WEE Protocol
for a Genomic-Specific Nutritional Plan

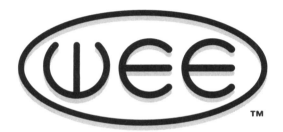

Work by the physician
to Examine and Evaluate

Work by the patient
to Educate themselves and
to Eat accordingly

Better Health In 120 Days

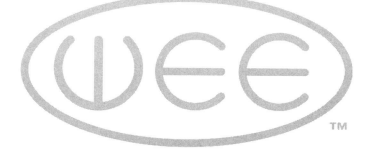

**Finding Answers with the WEE Protocol
for a Genomic-Specific Nutritional Plan**

Glen Aukerman, MD, DABFP, DABHM

The Wooster Book Company
Wooster ∾ Ohio
2012

The Wooster Book Company
where minds and imaginations meet
205 West Liberty Street
Wooster, Ohio • 44691
www.woosterbook.com

Neither the publisher nor the author is engaged in rendering professional advice or
services to the individual reader. The ideas, procedures, and suggestions contained
in this book are not intended as a substitute for consulting with your physician.
ALL MATTERS REGARDING YOUR HEALTH REQUIRE MEDICAL SUPERVISION.
Neither the author nor the publisher shall be liable or responsible for any loss or
damage allegedly arising from any information or suggestions in this book.

The recipes contained in this book are for illustration purposes only.
The author and publisher are not responsible for your specific health or allergy needs
which may require medical supervision. Neither the author nor the publisher is responsible
for any adverse reactions to the recipes contained in this book.

While the author has made every effort to provide accurate telephone numbers and
internet addresses at the time of publication, neither the publisher nor the author assumes any
responsibility for errors, or for changes that occur after publication. Further, neither the author nor
the publisher have any control over and do not assume any responsibility for authored or third-party
websites or their content.

Names of patients, where used, have been changed to protect the patients' privacy.

Printed and bound in the United States of America.

Book design by Jeff Hentosz

ISBN: 978-1-59098-012-5

Library of Congress Cataloging-in-Publication Data

Aukerman, Glen, 1940–
Better health in 120 days : finding answers with the wee protocol
for a genomic-specific nutritional plan / Glen Aukerman.
     p.   cm.
Includes bibliographic references.
ISBN 978-1-59098-012-5 (alk. paper)
1. Nutrition. 2. Diet. 3. Health. 4. Health promotion. I. Title.
QP141.A95 2011
613.2—dc23   2011029335

Contents

Inquiring Minds 1

Introduction to the WEE Protocol 9

Contributors to Modern Illness 25

Fixing It 51

Resources for Life—for the Rest of Your Life 101

Further Reading 115

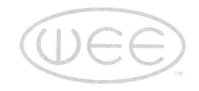

INQUIRING MINDS

Inquiring minds ask, "Why, out of all the really smart people in medicine and science who could have and probably should have created the WEE Protocol, did you do it? Why wasn't it discovered by the oncology experts, the endocrinology experts, the neurologists, or any of the other experts?"

I try, usually unsuccessfully, to give those asking this question a simplistic but true answer, explaining that the experts are likely distracted from finding creative answers by their years of being trained to think that the only acceptable solutions are ones backed by double-blind, random, controlled evidence (rat research, for example). Decades of researching a pharmaceutical solution to every problem has left many experts and pharmaceutical companies reluctant to consider creative options, like the WEE Protocol, that do not rely on traditional Western medications and practices.

It is important to note here that the WEE Protocol is also backed by research, as will be explained later in more detail.

If the resources offered by the pharmaceutical companies and traditional Western practitioners had actually worked for my more than 10,000 patients on their more than 32,000 visits with me, I doubt that I would have looked further and developed the protocol. We will never know, however, because those pharmaceutical and traditional Western approaches did not work for any of my patients or they would not have sought me out.

Upon further reflection, I must admit many of my early life experiences may have set the stage for me to develop the protocol. Because each of our lives is unique, my experience of searching, discovery, and then creation was unlikely to be duplicated by many others.

I was fortunate to be born the tenth child out of ten in a large farm family, where I learned to work every evening after school and every weekend on the farm and later in the restaurant business. I thereby developed the work ethic needed for medical school and residency.

Being born number ten of ten, and the seventh son of a seventh son, I was chosen early to be a doctor by my mother of Native American descent. She taught me her herbal remedies and always kept me focused on having a health care future.

Growing up on the farm allowed me to experience all aspects of food production, from eggs, to poultry, to sheep, to pork, to beef, to milking goats and dairy cattle. This in-depth experience gave me a unique perspective on a wide range of farm and food production issues. It later helped me to better understand how it was possible for the significant but subtle crop selection changes, occurring over the last fifty years in agribusiness, to create our nutrient-poor food supply of today. This background allowed me to discover why our food matters so much to our health status, from how we feel, think, and function, to how we get well or do not get well.

As it would happen, after medical school and residency, I was recruited to another rural Ohio area and went back to a farm to raise my family. I experienced a total of seven decades in and around agribusiness, minus the six years for medical school and residency when I had minimal opportunity to return to the farm. So understanding all about farming, the place where our nutrition begins, is big. No, it's more than big. It's huge! How our food is grown and produced directly impacts the nutrition we gain from it. The regulations and subsidies of the U.S. Department of Agriculture (USDA) and of the Food and Drug Administration (FDA) and other groups that impact agribusiness have directly affected the condition of our nutritional well-being. We will examine this in greater detail later.

I worked in my busy rural practice for 26.5 years in a western Ohio town of 1,100 people. After starting the practice, I expanded it with house calls, nursing home calls, and making rounds at the hospital. I eventually became the chief of staff of the regional 450-bed hospital when I was thirty-nine years of age. I made more than 536,000 patient visits, which consisted of about 336,000 office visits, about 56,000 nursing home visits, and about 145,000 hospital visits.

By that time, I was beginning to see how, where, when, and to whom diseases happen. At that career point, I was not aware of nutritional causes as being behind all the symptoms, abnormal tests, conditions, and diseases. We did think obesity could be from too much food, diabetes from too many carbohydrates, hypertension from too much salt, gout from too much alcohol and rich foods, but not to the extent that I now understand based on what I have since discovered.

Leadership opportunities in the Ohio and American Academies of Family Physicians led to my move from the rural practice to the Bureau of Health Professions in Washington, D.C. I enjoyed three years there as deputy director of quality assurance. My experience as a federal employee culminated with a three-month involvement with the Clinton Health Care Reform Initiative.

I then moved to West Virginia University (WVU), where as professor and chair of family medicine, I founded their integrative medicine program. That experience culminated in a national integrative medicine conference that I orchestrated at Cheat Lake in West Virginia.

In my WVU role, I also assumed leadership for Dr. Richard Iammarino's Healers-on-Call, a program in which a patient presented his or her unresolved problem or illness in a round table format to various community and campus healers, who proffered their solutions for the patient's consideration at no cost or obligation to the patient nor any liability to the healers.

The outcomes of this program were simply amazing! People would appear voluntarily at sessions with a one- to two-decade history of chronic pain and leave with multiple solutions they could begin at home. They would return to subsequent sessions free of the pain syndromes. They achieved the result by combining the several complementary alternative medicine (CAM) modalities offered at the prior session. Months later, they would show up again, stating that the pain had not come back.

Unfortunately, the program ended at WVU when I came to The Ohio State University, where we ran the program in 2005 and 2006. It is my hope to have the program up and running again.

For the last sixteen years, I have been at The Ohio State University. I began as Chair of Family Medicine, a largely administrative role, but by resigning the Chair position, I was able to move quickly back to my strength: taking care of patients. I became one-hundred percent in patient care at this Big Ten university with the appropriate teaching responsibilities.

For about two-thirds of this period, I was a consulting medical director to Nationwide Health Plans, part of Nationwide Inc., an insurance provider, until they outsourced their health-plan team. I was concurrently asked to be the interim medical director for The Ohio State University Health Plan. While working in this role with the plan's very capable staff, I was able to complete the plan's goal of ensuring that patients received coverage for complementary and alternative medical (CAM) services.

Both of these managed care experiences provided me with the knowledge and background in managed care to assist patients of integrative medicine in receiving the most from their insurance plans. To this date, all of my patients, if they have insurance, have been covered for the nutrigenomic work I do with them.

All these experiences further tempered my nutritional focus and my belief in the need for some new optimal health concepts.

Starting about eight years ago, I found myself spending my evenings and most weekends researching the amazing traditional health care dilemmas presented by my patients in office visits. I began in my off-duty time to explore the medical literature to identify solutions that might resolve their specific medical problems using my newly created nutrigenomic approach while reflecting on my approximately 536,000 rural patient care experiences and my sixty-some years of life experiences. I spent my evenings and weekends simply because there was not any time to research these problems during the busy flow of patient visits during my professional time. Many nights, I found my sleep interrupted by the many unanswered questions I had as to why my traditional medicine care did not succeed in resolving these patients' concerns.

In the process of analyzing these traditional health care dilemmas, I began to realize that the most puzzling problems were most often those that many of the very brightest medical specialists had failed to resolve. Was that because they were limited to traditional medicine's logic format, reductionism or because they could not improvise? Or because the doctor mistakenly thought the patient was getting better?

During that same time period, I was developing some new perceptions about these common yet unrecognized breaches in the nutrigenomic health/nutrition continuum. I can now recognize these breaks in nutrition underlying every symptom, abnormal lab result, and disease I had been working with on a daily basis, from autism and cancers to diabetes, fatigue, and pain. These nutritional deficiencies and food toxicities were giving rise to an immense need for reorientation and re-education about basic nutrition and how these breaks create and worsen most diseases, and yes, how to repair the breaks.

Before long, this effort was consuming every waking moment of my day. I was writing down possible treatments to respond to these breaks in the health/nutrition continuum, offering them to patients, and then writing them again. The results my patients reported made the long hours and hard work a very reasonable trade-off. Yes indeed, I was seeing better and better results in the patients coming back every day. They were telling me how they were getting their health—and their lives—back. These reports were a satisfying reward for my efforts. I care about my patients and devote my expertise to their healing by offering them options.

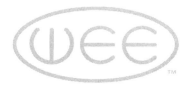

INTRODUCTION
TO THE WEE PROTOCOL

Have you ever walked into your doctor's office and said, "Doctor, what can you do to make me feel better?" If you have, you probably got a diagnosis and a prescription and were sent on your way.

But what would happen if you went to the doctor for help, only to find that the drugs didn't make any difference, or were too expensive, or had horrible side effects, or that you would have to take them for the rest of your life? What if the doctor said, "I'm sorry, but there's nothing else we can do."

Many of my patients find themselves in exactly this situation. They are desperately looking for solutions when traditional options no longer work.

Some six years ago, I created what has become a very successful protocol for applied nutrigenomics, which is the study of the relationship between one's diet and one's genes. Offered at over 32,000 patient visits, this protocol now appears to always result in predictable outcomes.

Nutrigenomics seeks to improve the functioning of one's genes through improved nutrition. It is based on the premise that what we eat directly impacts our genes and that when we eat according to what our genome requires, we can experience optimal health.

Since that time, I have observed in most if not all the subsequent patient visits, that the patients and their families coming to their first office visit share some amazingly similar characteristics. Many of the cases presented to me fell into several groups, all with nearly identical situations.

Group 1: About one-third of patients come with several unresolved symptoms, such as bloating, body aches, cloudy thinking, cold hands and feet, constipation, diarrhea, fatigue, getting up frequently at night to urinate, hair loss, headaches, heartburn, hives, impotence, mood problems, poor libido, poor sleep, problem complexions, rashes, recurring infections, restless legs, numbness, tingling, and the list goes on and on. These symptoms greet them when they open their eyes in the morning and are with them every moment of every day. Some get partially covered up by medicines but the symptoms never resolve and disappear in the traditional model.

Group 2: Another one-third of patients come with abnormal test results that they, their doctors, and their prescription drugs cannot clear completely or at all. These unresolved lab test results are particularly frustrating to the vast population of patients and their traditional doctors who rely on the golden idols of modern medicine, prescription drugs, to fix the problem. To their dismay, the tests may improve slightly but never clear completely and never stay cleared even with one, two, or three drugs. This is the case with the modern lipid profile. A bit of low HDL or high LDL or high triglycerides always remain. Even worse than the fact that the drugs do not do the job completely, patients are truly bothered to think they must take this medicine for asthma, depression, diabetes, erectile dysfunction, gastric reflux disorder, high blood pressure, heart disease, high cholesterol, itch, rash, sleeplessness, thyroid imbalance, and the list goes on, for the rest of their lives. As one patient said, "I will take these to my grave."

Group 3: The final one-third of patients come with diseases diagnosed as incurable, untreatable, or not responding to conventional treatment, alternative medicines, or to even the conjured-up concoctions found in holistic health and food outlets, most of which make patients' diseases and conditions worse. These diseases and conditions represent the full disease spectrum from A to Z, including ADD/ADHD, anxiety, asthma, Alzheimer's, and autism, and other terrible diseases, such as cancer, lupus, and multiple sclerosis. As with the first two groups, these patients are troubled to think they must take partially effective prescription medicines for the rest of their lives, while continuing to struggle with their chronic diseases and conditions. Many of this group say, "I am without hope if modern medicine cannot help my condition." Others report seeing only sadness in the eyes of their doctors and caregivers who are unable to help them.

Looking back at my more than 32,000 such visits with patients and their families representing more than 10,000 unique new patients and families over the last six years, I have observed certain things that now appear eerily consistent. Early on, I noticed that each patient and his or her family appeared to have failed in the quest for a cure of symptoms, abnormal lab tests, or diagnosed diseases and conditions.

I believe this is because neither the patient nor any of their doctors adequately understood the role the patient and family actively or passively played in contributing to their own illness. Their contribution came in the form of what I refer to as the nutrigenomic "dis-ease" path of least resistance. The term refers to the cascade of cellular processes in the body, set off by nutritional choices, which led these patients down the road to disease and dis-ease. By changing their nutritional choices, which I recognized as setting up the situations for illness, they can reverse the nutrigenomic "dis-ease" path of least resistance. The patients and their immediate and even extended families who joined them in making these changes then began to experience the beginnings of optimal health. Once they realized they were all ill to some extent, the sickest person in the family is no longer the token patient. The family becomes the patient.

I now recognize I coincidently started the "family process" by showing the others in the exam room that they are severely Vitamin B deficient (beriberi), or they have a latex rash on their chin, cheeks, ears or chest, or that they may even have thyroid nodules as well. This brings a new insight to light: a genetic phenomenon.

Now having developed and successfully implemented the protocol in more than 32,000 patient visits, early on I realized that what I was doing for and with patients and families required new educational tools and an orienting program. I have named this education and orientation process the WEE Protocol.

WEE stands for:

Work by the patient, based on

• Examination, ongoing monitoring, and
• Evaluation, and
• Extensive Education programming for patients and families

Prior to their initial office visit, all patients, their family members, and their support persons are introduced to the basic constructs of the WEE Protocol at a free community nutrigenomics class. Once they are aware of what is possible but what is required, they can be admitted to my nutrigenomic practice if they so desire. This book covers the principles presented in that class as well as offering a deeper explanation of the WEE Protocol.

The WEE Protocol is a set of rules and principles that I use with my patients to correct the defects in their ability to select appropriate nutrition based on their genotype. You might have heard the saying, "You are what you eat." Research is showing that this statement is true in ways we hadn't realized. Food and food components affect our individual physical characteristics more than we ever imagined. For those devoted to the WEE Protocol, being aware of what you eat is an ongoing lifetime of vigilant education and reeducation in ever continuing "E"s.

WEE Protocol
for a Genomic-Specific Nutritional Plan

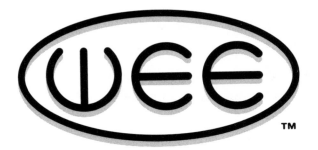

| Work by the physician to Examine and Evaluate | Work by the patient to Educate themselves and to Eat accordingly |

Think back to your high school biology class. You might remember hearing about your DNA, which resides in virtually every cell of your body (mature red blood cells lack a nucleus and DNA). Our DNA tells each cell its role by using genes, which instruct the cells to make various products, including proteins, to guide their processes.

All of our cellular processes can be related back to this basic chain of events carried out by DNA, genes, and proteins. When we say a gene is expressed, what is meant is that a section of DNA called a gene is transcribed into RNA and then translated into protein. Many, many factors influence gene expression, that is, which genes get transcribed and translated, which do not, and why, when, and how. This is why having the gene for something doesn't mean that you will ever express that gene. Which genes are expressed then directly impacts cellular process. This is how our genetic coding becomes manifest in our physical characteristics, in our capacities to function, and in our performance. Epigenetics is the study of how gene expression is impacted by factors other than those that directly impact the underlying DNA.

Research shows that the food we eat affects which proteins our genes express. Sometimes genes produce proteins that lead to optimal health, or homeostasis, meaning the body is in perfect balance. Other times, genes produce proteins that initiate illness or support an existing disease. The difference depends on what nutrients the genes receive.

This process explains how nutritional choices can impact your whole person. Your genes affect your cellular processes, which in turn affect bodily processes, which in turn affect your whole person. When a cellular process goes haywire, it can be traced back to the basic chain of events by DNA, genes, and proteins. Hence, foods or other elements that affect the directions given by our genes can lead to illness and disease or health and wellness. Understanding these connections is exciting stuff!

One group of proteins made by immune system cells, called cytokines, is drawing particular attention. Cytokines are involved in various types of cellular communication. They have been linked to inflammation, which leads to many of the chronic diseases and symptoms we mentioned earlier, and to the proliferation of cell growth connected to cancer.

One category of cytokine, the interleukins, is so named because of their role in communication among leukocytes, which are a type of white blood cell. White blood cells respond when our bodies are attacked by diseases or are wounded. Some interleukins stimulate the production of antibodies, while others induce the production of various types of blood cells. Interleukins and all cytokines are critical in immune function and disease processes.

Cancer researchers, doctors, pharmacists, and people in lab coats everywhere are working on ways to control cellular processes, especially the production of cytokines, in order to prevent, cure, and treat illness and disease. The WEE Protocol is equally interested in controlling cellular processes by correcting nutrigenomic defects to bring the body into homeostasis and leading to good health.

Nutrigenomics research is showing us that what we thought we knew about healthful nutritional choices isn't always matching what our genes need for optimal health. I have been offering these published research outcomes to the patients in my family practice for six years, for those more than 32,000 patient visits, and everyone has seen amazing results. Many patients who were pronounced terminally ill by the best oncologists and specialists have found their way to remission and some have returned to optimal health. Some have reported experiencing total remission of their conditions through the WEE Protocol.

When patients experience a disease, the problem is not simply that disease. Rather, it is specific set of nutrigenomic imbalances that create the symptoms and abnormal lab tests. These specific imbalances lead the patient's body to form a specific disease as a reaction. Getting "into" a disease is accidental, getting back out requires skill, education, and lifestyle changes that often encompass a lifetime.

The disease process is determined by what I call each individual's nutrigenetic "dis-ease path of least resistance." The term refers to the cascade of cellular processes leading to the expression of those cytokines responsible for the symptoms, including abnormal lab tests and resulting in specific diseases. The symptoms and lab tests point to toxicities, deficiencies, and/or excesses that affect the expression of genes in the patient's body. These toxicities, deficiencies, and excesses each accelerate—at a rate determined by the magnitude of their accumulation and their influence on the cytokines they produce—to push you along the nutrigenetic "dis-ease path of least resistance." By identifying and correcting those toxicities, deficiencies, and excesses, we can then correct the nutrigenetic "dis-ease path of least resistance."

I gain insight into the person's nutrigenetic "dis-ease path of least resistance" by doing the WEE Protocol Intake and the WEE Protocol 90/360 Lab Assessment, described in more detail later, to accurately predict the presence and severity of nutrigenomic abnormalities. Combining all of this information, I can calculate which deficiencies need replacements to begin getting the patient back on the road to better health.

The WEE Protocol Intake involves taking a detailed family history of symptoms, abnormal lab markers, and diseases. The "dis-ease path of least resistance" sets up the symptoms, abnormal lab tests, and subsequent diseases by closing down the patient's innate natural ability to prevent and correct disease, which is built into the incredible human genome. This natural ability can be blocked by toxic or excess substances piled upon deficiencies.

For patients who are adopted and come to the WEE Protocol Intake without a family history, I use their current symptoms, their abnormal lab markers, and their current and past medical history to validate which cytokines are being activated to create their unique problems. These tell me what the WEE Protocol needs to correct over the next 120 to 180 days if the person is to achieve optimal health.

Until now, these simple yet universal processes have been unknown or completely ignored by the patients, their families, and their doctors. From my observations of more than 32,000 patient visits, it appears that these symptoms, lab markers, and disease cascades, meaning all the cell processes that lead to a recognized or subtle disease, happen because patients have lost their natural genetic protection against the disease pathway that has been activated. All related disease formations in the same cytokine pathway accelerate unless I am able to stop them with the WEE Protocol. The protocol requires starting corrective actions to remove toxicities, rebalance the deficiencies, and reduce excesses.

Early in this work and patient by patient, I identified the elements of a personalized plan for each patient. Today, the WEE Protocol is very specific for each person's genetic markers, which can be identified from their current and past symptoms, abnormal lab results or markers, and medical history, with or without known family histories. Family history does, however, reinforce the accuracy of the assessment.

The WEE Protocol 90/360 Lab Assessment, given during the intake visit, confirms the patient's genetic markers and the corresponding cytokines functioning in the individual case. In my more than 32,000 patient visits, these highly specific lab results have corroborated the findings of my clinical exams, along with the patients' symptom diaries recording their specific symptoms, abnormal lab tests results, and their associated disease conditions. So far, the protocol has performed as predicted without exception. I noticed this degree of consistency during my first few thousand nutrigenomic patient encounters. Today's predictability still astonishes me, and I do this work six days out of seven most weeks. The results are just amazing!

This high degree of concurrence provides me with the confidence to predict almost precisely, within a one- or two-week period, when a symptom will begin to be alleviated and when most, if not all, abnormal lab tests will be removed—and this is within a 120-day time frame. If there is a lack of response on the part of the patient, typically he or she has not done the work of the Protocol.

One hundred and twenty days is the amount of time it takes to replace all of a patient's old red blood cells with new, fully loaded cells that are embedded with the nutrient protection they were intended to have naturally. One hundred and twenty days is the time needed to return patients' cells to a state that existed before our foods became empty of nutrients and too complex, our water became devoid of essential minerals, and alien foods were introduced onto our dining tables and into our meal plans.

Since this nutrigenetic path of least resistance is present in each family member, it is important to have the entire family participate in the WEE Protocol. First, all family members will benefit, and second, the patient becomes terminal when abnormal processes become fixed and no longer respond to nutrigenomic treatment. In my more than 32,000 patient visits, this has only occurred when the patient or family terminates the WEE Protocol, either on purpose, by negligence, or by accident. From my observations, termination unfortunately results in death in about six to eight weeks in patients thought to be terminal. Death usually occurs in a low calcium, magnesium, and Vitamin D state.

Early in my observations, I was able to get to the real cause of the patient's problem: their food-water-gene mismatch. Then, by re-educating the patient and the patient's family about the concepts and solutions and by removing or correcting the problems, I would help them see some amazing results.

During this time, I also realized some patients were losing to their diseases because they were being distracted from their healthful program. To correct this, I developed WEE Protocol educational programming to better protect patients from their well-intentioned yet misinformed friends, neighbors, health care workers and providers. All of these "helpers" offered old ideas with no new science behind them and no lab markers to document positive change. These helpers therefore had no chance to restore the patient's health. Instead, they distracted the entire patient-family-support team just long enough for the patient to lose his or her tenuous grip on life. For very frail or ill patients, often there is no "re-do" if they lose a valuable six to eight weeks before reaching optimal health and remission of their disease is therefore not likely.

All symptoms and diseases can now be viewed as the result of patients' poor choices, or lack of choices, in terms of food, water, and their environment. Sad but true, these choices, whether made actively or passively, have their impact on the patient and the patient's family. Before attending the educational programs, most patients and their families do not know the effect of the choices they are making. Now, the WEE Protocol programming educates patients and families so that they understand their choices and are able to make better ones. The difference is as pronounced as night and day.

I uncovered these principles by doing extensive research in peer-reviewed, evidence-based, nutritional and medical literature while trying to recover the health of a desperate patient.

PEER REVIEWED means each journal article, before it is published, is reviewed by a panel of experts in the subject area. These experts verify that the study described in the article was conducted using high-quality procedures. If an article does not meet the approval of the experts, it is not published, though this may not be true of all health advice that is out there.

EVIDENCE BASED means that scientific proof exists to document the accuracy of the principle being discussed. These evidence-based principles are mostly unknown to the majority of physicians, dietitians, and nutritionists. The practitioners can learn about the principles by reading the research, as I did, and by caring enough to go the extra mile for the patient in trouble who seeks answers, then improvising to make improvements happen.

In 2005, my entire forty-one-year medical practice changed when a young woman named Lisa came into my office with the desire to stay alive long enough to see her newborn child enter grade school. She had just been given sixty days to live by her oncologist. This is the patient who launched me on the applied nutrigenomic approach to medicine. We learned a great deal together, and many after her have benefited from her heartfelt request. I have summarized her story here, but you can read more details in the full case study found in the Fixing It section.

She committed, as did I, to work on the program that became the foundation of the WEE Protocol. As I followed her case, I noticed that some things in her lab work were improving with the food changes and the supplemental fish oil I recommended. After six months on my new protocol, she was taken off her cancer medications and hypertensive chemotherapy by the oncologist. She was told that she was in remission. She was elated! She could hope to see her child enter school.

Her health blossomed, but I continued to watch her metabolic markers from time to time. Today, I continue to be surprised that most internists, oncologists, and even endocrinologists do not watch for complications in patient cases or try to prevent them. Sadly, her cancer returned, and her oncologist enrolled her in a clinical trial that took her off my protocol. She died nine months after quitting the protocol from low levels of magnesium.

One of the sad but important lessons I learned from this first patient is that terminally ill patients who begin to show improvement on the protocol will relapse and deteriorate quickly if they stop the protocol in its exact form.

Today, when I see a new patient, although he or she is often depressed by the diagnosis, I am usually able to get him or her and the family excited by the fact that together, we will soon have lab results indicating new opportunities to be healthy again. We will know, within a few hours or a few days at the most, based on my 90/360 lab profile, why the patient has been feeling off for years but could never put a finger on what exactly was wrong.

Then, when we get together in my office, we will begin to discover the exact underlying cause for their illnesses, symptoms, abnormal labs, or diseases. Together, we can take some precise actions that will predictably reverse these diseases and prevent them from recurring. We can even prevent a disease's rapid progression since we now have a wide range of lab markers that indicate, and validate, the effectiveness of the patient's compliance with the WEE Protocol. There is no longer a reason for depression brought on by a new diagnosis to linger once realistic hope begins.

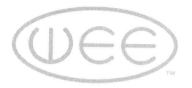

CONTRIBUTORS
TO MODERN ILLNESS

Those on the WEE Protocol are systematically looking for answers, learning what changes in their dietary patterns are necessary, and living those changes daily. Through applied nutrigenomics, we make illness-to-health changes relating to every symptom, condition, disease, and nonoptimal lab result by correcting our water-food-genome mismatches. My patients report that these water-food-genome solutions have worked miracles in their lives.

I am now beginning to believe that, until the use of the WEE Protocol, we in traditional medicine have failed completely in curing any metabolic disease by limiting ourselves to the diagnosis of the disease, then looking for a drug or procedure as the ultimate treatment. By treating only the symptoms or labs associated with the disease with drugs, such as ACE inhibitors for hypertension, diabetes drugs for elevated HgbA1c, statins for lipids, and mood drugs for situational stress and depression, we often remain oblivious to the real causes of diseases: the water/food/genome mismatch.

Whatever the symptom, abnormal lab marker, or disease, when I research modern medical literature on *www.pubmed.gov*, I find information about the cytokines that trigger the problems as well as cytokines that quiet them down. *PubMed.gov* is a Web source created by the National Institutes of Health, and the U.S. National Library of Medicine, where the discoveries of scientific research are made accessible to the public.

Based on my years of experience and my research in relation to my practice, many of today's health issues appear to be the result of an epidemic of silent food intolerance that has exploded in the population since 1950. We find support for this idea in that humans did not develop the majority of modern diseases until the following occurred:

- We added genomically alien and plant-oil-based foods including seeds and nuts to our ancestral diet.
- We created metabolic confusion in our body's immune system with too much food variety and "fad" diets.
- We began eating a diet high in omega-6 fatty acids contained in plant oil that stimulates excess cytokines without the correct, natural omega-3 reserve to provide balance.
- We lost essential minerals from our drinking water.
- We began consuming fruits and vegetables deficient in six essential nutrients.

- We developed increased latex sensitivities as a result of our eating newly available foods containing latex-like proteins and inhaling latex fumes generated by tires on our busy roads.
- Artificial chemicals, including monosodium glutamate (MSG), artificial sweeteners, food coloring, and preservatives became prevalent in all processed foods.
- Microwaves created new chemical toxins in foods from plastic containers, especially those used for sealed meals.

These factors, combined with the emotional and physiological stresses of modern life, have led to a society that is sick to the core. We are malnourished, exhausted, dissatisfied, and unfulfilled. All the while, each advance that promises to resolve our problems leads to another dysfunction. At the core of this dysfunction is the disruption of our water-food-genome continuum.

Our difficulties began about five hundred years ago when people and foods began to move across continents in an unprecedented manner, disturbing the prime-absolute for human health, which lies in maintaining our historically perfectly matched water-food-genome continuum. The continuum had existed uninterrupted since our beginnings as a result of an absence of any intervening events or factors including long-distance travel and food shipments.

Then, starting in the 1950s, deep-seated changes in our basic food and water supplies occurred as a byproduct of science and other innocent-looking but health-reducing phenomena. These included heightened exposure to genomically alien foods, increased exposure to latex-like proteins, water depleted of minerals, increased plant oil

1492	• Opening of the world trade routes introduces alien foods to human societies • Corn, potatoes, tomatoes, and peanuts are introduced to eastern hemisphere populations • Wheat is introduced to western hemisphere populations
1700s	• Movement of peoples to new food environments including Europeans to North America as industry developed • Africans and Asians moved to North American food environments
1909	• Rubber developed for tires which will lead to latex sensitivity by 1979 • Soy oil pressed for first time which is introduced into food production by World War I
1940s	• Foods and technology distributed by WWII leading to alien foods becoming widely available • Multiple sclerosis first noted in 1943
1950s	• Crop selection leads to six nutrient deficiencies in forty-three garden crops in the United States and eventually worldwide • Latex-like proteins in foods first eaten by humankind which is also a problem due to inhaled rubber from tires
1970s	• Softened, city, and bottled water introduced in rich-world cities • Food additives expanded to all humankind
1990s	• Alien foods marketed as healthful along with the illusion that food variety is beneficial • Acid reflux, fibromyalgia, osteopenia epidemics due to loss of minerals in food and in the water supply
2005	• OSU Center for Integrative Medicine opens • First patient placed on WEE Protocol for nutrigenomics
2010	• Over 32,000 patient visits on WEE Protocol • Epigenetics becomes a protocol option

FIGURE 2. *The nutrigenomic history of modern diseases from 1940 to 2010 shows how many factors have contributed to modern diseases and the nutrient-gene mismatch.*

consumption, and nutrient deficiencies in our fruits and vegetables. A timeline reflecting these changes appears in Figure 2.

The next section gives an overview of each of these contributors to modern disease and how the WEE Protocol works to correct them.

Water

You have probably heard that it is important to drink plenty of water. You might know that humans can survive only days without water. Why is water so important? It is critical for all body functions and processes from digestion and circulation to cellular communication and energy transformations.

Before modern civilizations began processing and bottling water, our water contained important minerals that contributed to health: essential calcium, magnesium, and potassium. After industrialization, the need to supply clean water to large populations led to public utilities and water treatment systems. These water treatment systems, created with the intention of protecting health and ensuring uniform taste in water, unintentionally caused new health problems.

Since 1950, we have replaced hard well water that is rich in magnesium, potassium, and calcium with magnesium-, potassium-, and calcium-depleted softened and bottled water. The depletion of these key minerals from the water is a major contributing cause for arthritis, asthma, constipation, diabetes, fatigue, gastric reflux disorder, headaches, insomnia, metabolic syndrome, osteopenia, osteoporosis, panic disorders, and colon, esophageal, ovarian, and prostate cancers (per the National Institutes of Health).

By the 1960s, softened and treated water in the cities was depleted of its mineral content. In the 1980s, many began drinking bottled water, and the belief that water from the tap was unhealthy was perpetuated. The popularity of water treated by reverse osmosis in the 1990s further depleted the mineral content. Today, we are left with empty water that fails to support our health. Empty water enters the body but water with essential minerals leaves the kidneys and sweat glands.

Food and Gluten Intolerances

Intolerance to gluten and other foods results from the regular introduction of genomically alien foods on a scale that overwhelms the human immune system. If your ancestors have not had at least 10,000 years of eating experience with a food, it should be considered genomically alien or outside your genome.

Since coming to the New World in 1492, European Americans have been exposed to numerous genomically alien foods, such as corn, green peppers, peanuts, potatoes, and tomatoes. Since 1492, Asian and Native Americans have been introduced to gluten. In Iran, it has been only 2,500 years since humans first ate wheat and a similar period of time with maize in Central and South American.

With five hundred years of world travel and immigration leading to an increasingly global society, the genes of the human race have become mixed. It is no longer so simple to say, my family is mostly of European decent, so I should eat this and avoid that. Each individual's genes are unique. Therefore, the WEE Protocol takes the family history and ancestry into account but bases diagnoses of food intolerances on individual lab tests and symptoms. Each person's response to the WEE Protocol is validated for their genome through systematic correlation of abnormal and suboptimal lab results.

Although dairy products are often blamed for many symptoms, humans have had experience with dairy for about 6,000 years. I have found that my patients' symptoms are most often from the underlying gluten problems, not from dairy products. Gluten is a protein found in many grains. The most commonly eaten grains in North America that contain gluten are wheat, barley, and rye. New research has shown that *avenin* in oats is gluten-like and soy, sorghum, buckwheat, and millet test positive for gluten as well. Once patients resolve the damage from the underlying gluten problem, they resume eating dairy with no adverse effects.

By now, you may have heard of people who eat gluten free and may even know someone who is on a gluten-free diet. You might even have heard of celiac disease, an autoimmune disorder triggered by consuming gluten. Celiac disease is a serious illness in which the immune system attacks the lining of the small intestine. It can lead to bloating, diarrhea, constipation, infertility, intestinal lymphoma cancer, and malnourishment, to name a few effects. The National Institutes of Health (NIH) estimates that up to one in 133 people have been diagnosed with celiac disease, and that ninety-five percent of people affected are undiagnosed, the tip-of-an-iceberg of gluten-based disease.

The Real Facts about Flax

Flaxseed and flaxseed (linseed) oil are rich sources of the essential fatty acid alpha-linolenic acid, a building block for omega-3 fatty acids in most animals. However, in humans, only 0.2–8 percent can be converted to the healthful EPA/DHA in the liver versus its presence in rats. These animals were the original research subjects showing effective conversion. The forty-fold difference in conversion rates appears to be due to human diets that are high in omega-6 fatty acids which lowers conversions. Regardless of the reason, while the amount of ALA believed to be converted to DHA in humans remains controversial, with some studies showing only small amounts, it is prudent to avoid these potential sources of non-convertible ALA.

Patients should avoid flax or flax oil if they have prostate cancer, breast cancer, uterine cancer, or endometriosis, or if they have a history of acute/chronic diarrhea, bowel obstruction, esophageal stricture, gastrointestinal stricture, ileus, irritable bowel syndrome, or diverticulitis/inflammatory bowel disease.

Caution is given to those with a history of a bleeding disorder, who take drugs that cause bleeding risk, such as anticoagulants, or nonsteroidal anti-inflammatories, such as aspirin, warfarin, or ibuprofen, as well as those with asthma, diabetes, high triglyceride levels, mania, or seizures. Avoid flax and flax oil if pregnant or breastfeeding.

I do not recommend that any of my patients consume flax products. The risks, and the contribution to omega-6 toxicity outweigh any benefits.

- NO FLAX -

The symptoms of individuals with gluten intolerance or gluten sensitivity can mirror those of people with celiac disease; however, a study published in March 2011 in the journal *BMC Medicine*, outlines the clinical difference between the pathology of celiac disease and the pathology of gluten sensitivity. Differentiating between the two is a topic of current interest to researchers studying gluten-related bowel disorders. The core difference appears to be the eliciting of an autoimmune reaction. Individuals with celiac disease experience an autoimmune response when they consume gluten. The symptoms experienced by those with gluten sensitivity are not always caused by an autoimmune reaction. However, it is important for both groups to maintain a strictly gluten-free diet which can be monitored by periodic anti-gluten lab tests.

In about ninety-five percent of my patients, I have observed gluten-induced bowel damage at levels significant enough to generate severe autoimmune or chemical sensitivity diseases. Consuming gluten-containing grains increases the severe deficiencies of calcium, magnesium, and trace minerals, plus Vitamins A, D, E, B, B-12, and K, as a result of small bowel malabsorption caused by gluten-induced bowel damage on top of what is missing in all forty-three garden crops, and in our water.

Bowel damage from gluten begins to heal once gluten is removed from the diet. Removing all sources of gluten and gluten-like proteins can be difficult. Cross-contamination in inherently gluten-free grains is a widespread problem, which you can read more about in the side bar. Oats, while previously thought to be gluten free or to be at the most contaminated from wheat in the farmer's field or factory processing, have now been documented to have avenin which acts as gliadin to destroy the small bowel lining of sensitive people such as celiacs. But even when they are free from gluten cross-contamination, some people with celiac disease do not tolerate them. I no longer recommend that my patients consume oats if they are sensitive to gluten. As research continues to provide more information, we may discover more gluten-like proteins that cause damage.

Gluten Cross-Contamination of Gluten-Free Grains

Many grains were considered to be inherently gluten free. That is, they are not direct relatives of wheat and do not have the same protein components. Such grains are often grown near wheat, however, and processed in facilities that also handle wheat or other gluten-containing grains.

In a study published in June 2010 in the "Journal of the American Dietetic Association," researchers tested the gluten content of inherently gluten-free grains and flours that were not labeled gluten free. Their research showed that 59 percent of the products tested contained less than five ppm (parts per million) of gluten. Some products, 32 percent of those tested, contained more than twenty ppm of gluten and 41 percent had less than five ppm. These products would not be permitted to carry a gluten-free label under the

Plant Oils

Historically, humans are believed to have eaten a diet that contained a roughly 1:1 balance of omega-3 and omega-6 fatty acids, which are dietary fats contained in almost every food, including fruits and vegetables. Omega-3 and omega-6 fatty acids cannot be synthesized by the body, and both are important for development and immune function, therefore are essential oils for humans.

proposed FDA rules for gluten-free labeling. Grains tested included amaranth, buckwheat, corn, millet, rice, sorghum, and soy with the buckwheat, millet, sorghum, and soy containing large amounts of gluten-like readouts.

It is important for people following a gluten-free diet to consider the risk of eating what was previously thought to be inherently gluten-free grains regardless of gluten-free labeling. Some, but not all, potentially contaminated foods carry an allergen warning statement. It is my experience that corn, potato, and rice are the safest, though inroads have been made to keep more inherently gluten-free grains safe. Today they cannot be considered safe. However, as you will read, not all gluten-free grains are free of other contributors to modern illness.

When the balance of omega-3 to omega-6 becomes too heavily tilted toward omega-6, however, inflammation and inflammatory diseases result. The percentage of long-chain omega-6 fatty acids stored in an individual's body is determined by his or her food choices. NIH-supported research shows that in countries where the percentage of long-chain omega-6 fatty acids consumed is lower, the incidence of heart attack related deaths is also lower, as is illustrated in Table 1. Note that long-chain fatty acids have stronger effects than short-chain fatty acids. The difference is caused by more or fewer carbon atoms making up the chain.

Dietary Omega-6 Fatty Acids and Heart Attack Deaths				
	Inuit	Japan	Mediterranean	United States
Percentage of long-chain omega-6 fatty acids*	<25	47	58	78
Heart attack deaths per 100,000 people	<25	50	90	200

* This percentage is representative of the omega-6 to omega-3 balance; viz, 50% would be roughly equivalent to a 1:1 omega-6 to omega-3 ratio. Data obtained from: *http://efaeducation.nih.gov*

There are three forms of omega-3 fatty acids found in food: α-linolenic acid (ALA), eicosapentaenoic acid (EPA), and docosahexaenoic acid (DHA). EPA and DHA are linked to reduced inflammation and reduced risk of coronary artery disease and associated factors. ALA has not been shown to have the same effect as EPA and DHA in humans. In fact, research has shown that humans have a difficult time converting ALA to EPA/DHA (converting 0.2% for omnivores to 8% for carnivores). Thus, ALA contributes to the omega-6 toxicity associated with high amounts of plant oils in the Western diet. The section with helpful resources contains figures showing the increases in cytokine pathways that result when humans eat dietary omega-3 or omega-6 fatty acids.

Starting in 1909, the food industry began to incorporate ever increasing amounts of omega-6 plant oils—first soybean oil, then a cascade of other plant oils—into the increasingly complex food base. New evidence from research in the last five years shows that the three essential dietary oils, omega-3, omega-6, and omega-9, need to be in a 1:1:1 ratio for optimal health but have now been estimated to be 1:30:1.

Omega-9 comes from trees (olive oil). Olive oil is the only plant oil that I recommend to my patients. Even then, it should be used sparingly. Changing this ratio from 1:1:1 leads to most modern chronic diseases, such as cancers, depression, diabetes, heart disease, hypertension, obesity, plus acute conditions of anxiety, fatigue, panic disorder, and pain.

Since 2004, many physicians have suggested that their patients eat more omega-6-laden corn-fed poultry and farmed fish, flax, nuts, seeds, soy, and chickpeas (also known as garbanzo beans). They recommend avoiding the more healthful beef, pork, lamb, eggs, and butter, which in comparison are lower in omega-6 fatty acids. Without reading the latest peer-reviewed, evidence-based nutritional research literature, neither patients, their doctors, nor health food stores can know, or would have known, that the foods and products ladened with the omega-3 ALA, seeds such as flax and soy, and all white meats, are processed by the human body as if they were omega-6 plant oil and are contributing to the problem.

Ingestion of these foods further contributes to patients' omega-6-based, plant-oil-related symptoms, abnormal lab tests, and disease processes. Many health food stores and even doctors have marketed many of these foods, specifically those high in ALA, saying they are "good for you" because they are rich in omega-3 fatty acids. You might have heard that nuts and flax in particular are heart healthy and anti-inflammatory. However, nuts, flax, and many other health products containing seeds, soy, and chickpeas have minimal EPA and DHA and are extremely high in ALA. Thus, they add to the omega-6 toxicity and push you further away from your health target.

Many gluten-free "grains" and "alternative flours" that are being marketed and produced for the growing gluten-free population are high in omega-6 fatty acids. For example, teff is an inherently gluten-free grain that is really a seed. Like all seeds, it is high in omega-6 fatty acids. Nut flours are also prevalent in gluten-free products. It is important to read product labels and do your research before eating a new food. As we continue to learn, all that is marketed as healthy is not necessarily so. (See *http://efaeducation.nih.gov*)

Food choices that increase omega-6 toxicity and imbalance cause the massive inflammatory problems associated with most modern diseases and immune disorders, including cancers. Foods that contribute to omega-6 fatty acid toxicity include the following:

- corn-fed poultry and farm-raised fish
- nuts, nut oils, and nut flours
- seeds, seed oils, and butters (including flax)
- soy and soy derivatives
- chickpeas (also called garbanzo beans) and hummus
- granola that contains nuts, seeds, and plant oils
- corn oil and corn additives

Food choices that contain a positive balance of DHA and EPA omega-3 fatty acids have been shown to reduce inflammation and decrease the effects of the Western diet. Foods that contribute to omega-3:omega-6 balance include the following:

- cruciferous vegetables (e.g., broccoli, brussels sprouts, and cauliflower)
- leafy greens (e.g. lettuce, spinach, and kale)
- squash (e.g., pumpkin, winter squash, and zucchini)
- green and wax beans
- kidney and pinto beans
- wild-caught salmon
- shrimp and crab
- sardines and tuna pack in water, not oil
- papaya and papaya nectar*
- mangos*
- cantaloupe and honeydew*
- some cheeses (i.e., Gouda, Parmesan, Romano, and Roquefort)

The items marked with an asterisk (*) should be ripened naturally on the tree or plant or avoided as they contain latex, which will be discussed in further detail later. Most supermarket versions

Poor Memory and Impaired Cognitive Functions

Charlotte: My "Why Can't I Get My Mind Together" Patient

My "Why Can't I Get My Mind Together" patient Charlotte sat depressed and worn-looking in the exam room chair, clothing in disarray, hair a mess but appeared clean enough. I said, "Hello, I am Dr. Aukerman. What can I do to help?" Her first words were, "Why can't I get my mind together?"

Over the next few minutes, this patient revealed that she was homeless and living out of her car. She had dropped out of her master's degree program because her mind was not clear. She could not string together the necessary thoughts to make sense of her work anymore. She denied drug use, so why would her memory and other cognitive functions work so poorly? Additionally, she was not sleeping because she was disturbed by multiple nighttime urinations.

My "Why Can't I Get My Mind Together" patient was fortunate to be on a Medicaid prescription drug plan that allowed for a multivitamin, high-potency vitamin B complex, magnesium oxide tablets, and calcium carbonate with vitamin D. Unfortunately, her Medicaid plan would not provide the fish oil needed to complete the first stage of balancing her excess in omega-6 plant oils. I gave her a $10 bill for her first bottle of high-potency fish oil. She returned the change, $2.87, to my medical assistant.

By the time Charlotte returned for her next visit, I had spent most of my hours after work and on the weekend trying to understand the immunologic mechanisms at work in the absorption and replacement of micronutrients such as the B-complex vitamins and minerals such as magnesium and calcium. I studied the research explaining the effect of compensating with the high-potency omega-3 fish oil to balance the excess of 20-30 times in omega-6 plant oils now apparent in all our new processed foods. I took into consideration our new awareness of the naturally occurring latex in avocados, bananas, celery, figs, kiwis, and eight other fruits and vegetables.

When Charlotte returned in another month for her third visit, she related how she had been feeling so much better, she was able to develop a meaningful relationship with a man and so had moved out of her car. In addition, she had re-entered her master's program in education. Now she could afford her own fish oil while Medicaid furnished the rest of her supplements. In three months, Charlotte completed her master's program and secured a teaching position in a public school system ... all for $7.13, from my point of view.

Further research indicated that Charlotte no doubt was depressed and cognitively dysfunctional from a multifaceted deficiency disorder, combined with her consumption of foods with excess plant oil foods. All these factors contributed to her situational depression. To date, she is still employed in the public school system as a teacher, is still in the meaningful relationship, and is happier.

will have been picked green and imported. Frozen or canned may be safe, as they are more likely to have been picked when naturally ripe and processed at a plant near where they were grown.

A complete list of recommended foods, their omega content, and other nutritional information is found in the section with helpful resources.

Nutrient-Deficient Fruits and Vegetables

Since 1950, all forty-three fruits and vegetables familiar in the United States have become deficient in six essential nutrients. In 2004, the *Journal of the American College of Nutrition* published a study confirming that forty-three garden crops had become less nutritious since 1950. Traditionally grown and organics were both included in the study. It was found that even the organics were less nutritious now than they were sixty years ago. As reported, this change, which was unexpected and unintentional, is due to crop selection favoring the farmers' productivity (and not to be confused with genetic modification).

The study also reported that our forty-three fruits and vegetable were never tested for their nutrient content by the USDA until 1999, and then they were all found to be deficient in six essential nutrients. With all forty-three foods being nutrient deficient, and with the National Institutes of Health reporting that water-based products and softened city and bottled water are severely mineral deficient, especially in magnesium and calcium, labels stating that products are alive, fast, slow, free-range, fresh, packaged, and whole matter little. *Empty equals empty, no matter how you label, promote, or process it. And toxic equals toxic even if labeled gluten-free today.*

The study examined protein, calcium, phosphorous, iron, ribo-flavin (a B vitamin), and vitamin C content of these forty-three fruits and vegetables with the following findings:

- protein: 6 percent decline, which leads to protein-calorie malnutrition
- calcium: 16 percent decline, which leads to osteoporosis, osteopenia, and muscle and bone weakness
- phosphorus: 9 percent decline, which leads to osteoporosis, osteopenia, and muscle and bone weakness
- iron: 15 percent decline, which leads to anemia, fatigue, and growth problems in children

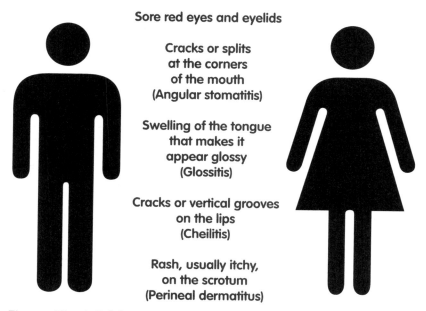

Figure 3. *Vitamin B deficiency signs, symptoms, and problems visible to your doctor in the examination room.*

- riboflavin: 38 percent decline, which leads to beriberi symptom complex manifesting as chronic fatigue and irritability
- Vitamin C: 15 percent decline, which leads to immune deficiency disorders and lowered resistance to infections

The shift from the use of magnesium-rich fertilizers from animals fed on grass to mineral-deficient commercial fertilizers for food crops led to loss of magnesium in the soil. This increased deficits of magnesium in the current grocery-based food supply. The problem was compounded by a shift of Western populations' produce source from the magnesium-rich fruits and vegetables grown in the home garden to the grocery-based, magnesium-deficient produce.

I have found that most of my patients arrive with some level of vitamin and mineral deficiencies. From the time I first meet a patient, there are some vitamin B deficiency signs and symptoms that have become obvious. Figure 3 shows some of the most visible.

Latex-like Proteins

When ingested by humans, these latex-like proteins suppress the immune system, enhance pain in those with sensitivities, and reduce the body's resistance to cancer for forty-eight to seventy-two hours. Autoimmune reactions to latex-like proteins include chemical sensitivity conditions, immune system depression, increased pain, fibromyalgia, anxiety, depression, and poor quality of sleep.

B Complex Vitamins and Their Deficiency Signs	
Vitamin Dose Needed	**Deficiency Signs and Symptoms**
Thiamin (B1), 100 mg	Beriberi rashes, polyneuritis, PMS, Wernicke-Korsakoff Syndrome, restless leg syndrome
Riboflavin (B2), 100 mg	Dermatitis, cheilosis, angular stomatitis, lack of growth
Niacin, 100 mg Nicotinic acid Nicotinamide	Dermatitis, dementia, pellagra with diarrhea
Vitamin B6, 100 mg Pyridoxine Pyridoxamine	Nasolabial seborrhea, glossitis, periperal neuropathy, epileptiform convulsions in infants
Pantothenic acid, 100 mg	Fatigue, sleep disturbances, impaired coordination, nausea
Biotin, 100 mg	Fatigue, depression, nausea, dermatitis, muscular pains

Latex-like proteins occur naturally in a variety of foods, such as avocados, bananas, celery, figs, kiwi, and out-of-season stone fruits, such as apricots, cherries, nectarines, peaches, and plums, as well as other out-of-season fruits, melons, tomatoes, and vegetables that are shipped from other regions. They also occur in most so-called "live" health food products, which contain components extracted from fruits or vegetables before they were fully vine, tree, or plant ripened. Shipping fruits and vegetables across regions and live health food products gained popularity since the 1960s as a way to get more fresh fruits and vegetables out of season and out of region. This now contributes to bringing alien food to our genome, many containing latex.

The practice of shipping such foods to regions where they are out of season has expanded to the point where most people are eating latex-laden foods on a regular basis, often daily. This might not have been a problem except for the fact that beginning in the 1920s, people became increasingly exposed to latex proteins from rubber compounds as fumes from rubber automobile tires generated on our roads. It became a health problem in the 1980s when the pollution from rubber tire fumes became great enough to sensitize large portions of our populations to latex proteins in the rubber compounds used in tires.

When inhaled, latex proteins produce an immune system sensitization that causes a chemical cross-sensitivity reaction to the latex-like proteins in food. Cross-sensitivity to latex-like proteins as a result of exposure to auto tire fumes was first reported in academic journals by the National Institute of Environmental Health (NIEH) in 1979.

Some of the common foods with defined cross-reactivity to latex are almonds, apples, avocados, bananas, carrots, celery, chestnuts, hazelnuts, kiwis, melons, papayas, pears, raw potatoes, stone fruits, and tomatoes. Foods with less well-defined cross-reactivity to latex are citrus fruits, coconuts, figs, grapes, mangoes, passion fruit, peanuts, peppers, pineapples, and Ugli fruit. New Class 2 food allergies now extend these principles to other plant products, including prolamins.

Cross-reactivity is a reaction between an antigen and an antibody that was generated against a different antigen with similar properties. **Cross sensitivity** is the sensitivity to a substance that predisposes an individual to sensitivities to other substances that have a similar chemical structure.

Physicians often have recommended that their patients consume foods laden with naturally occurring latex-like protein, especially avocados, bananas, celery, figs, and kiwis. They do this in order to increase potassium levels despite the fact that evidence-based research shows these foods increase latex reaction in latex-sensitive people. As mentioned previously, the shipping of these foods over long distances allows people to buy them in the grocery store out of season. This distribution has so expanded that most people eat latex-containing foods daily furthering their multiple-chemical sensitivities.

According to the *Annals of Allergy*, cited in the further reading section, up to half of latex-sensitive patients show allergic reactions to fruits such as avocados, bananas, kiwis, papayas, and peaches. These plants contain the same proteins that are allergens in latex. People with fruit allergies should warn physicians before undergoing procedures, as these fruit allergies may actually cause an anaphylactic reaction if the patient comes in contact with latex gloves or other latex-containing items, even IV tubing.

Artificial Chemicals

In an attempt to make food healthier and cheaper, the food industry has come up with some fabulous fakes that the popular health culture has claimed as its own. How many health and fitness magazines encourage readers to use sugar substitutes to lead a healthier lifestyle?

Monosodium glutamate (MSG), sugar substitutes such as aspartame, saccharin, and sucralose, and all of the other food additives that have become an accepted part of the Western diet must all be processed through the liver. When you consume a diet high in food additives, you increase stress on the liver. In addition, many people have chemical sensitivities to many food additives. This is why many people find that they feel better and healthier on a simpler diet of whole and minimally processed foods.

MSG has been associated with a host of health issues, including impaired glucose tolerance, impaired liver function, inflammation, insulin resistance, and obesity. Excessive MSG consumption has also been linked with gastritis and gastric and duodenal ulcers. MSG has been implicated in "Chinese Restaurant Syndrome," which is a reaction to foods containing MSG (e.g., hot dogs and Chinese food). The reactions reported by the NIH for this syndrome include chest pain, flushing, headache, numbness or tingling around the mouth, pressure or swelling in the face, sweating, and death.

Artificial chemicals have also been introduced into the Western diet by the increased use of microwaves for cooking food. Research has shown that exposing plastics to microwaves increases the rate at which the plastic degrades. This causes leaching of toxic chemicals into the food within seconds to minutes.

Research has also shown that the way food is cooked matters. Food is chemically altered when cooked, depending on the cooking method, such as boiling, frying, roasting, and microwaving. You might have heard that boiling broccoli in water is a less healthful way to cook it than steaming it. This is because more nutrients are lost in the cooking water during boiling than are lost when broccoli is steamed above water. There are methods of cooking that can improve the nutritional qualities of certain foods, whereas other cooking methods can degrade nutritional components and even produce toxic components.

Heating or cooking in plastic containers has been shown to cause the plastic to break down. Most plastics release harmful chemicals that can leach into your food when used for food storage, for heating, or for cooking food.

I recommend that my patients limit the use of the microwave as much as possible. If microwaving is unavoidable, do not microwave food in plastic containers. Glass containers are preferable for heating foods in the microwave and for food storage.

For those readers interested in reading some of the scientific journal articles described as found during my research, please refer to the Further Reading section.

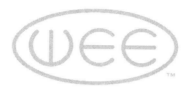

FIXING IT

Now that we know what is wrong with our food supply and the health information that the media provides, how do we go about fixing the problem?

Whenever patients and their family supporters adhere to the simple, well-defined nutrigenomic WEE Protocol and do their assigned homework, they are amazed at the health improvements they achieve. Whoever distracts them from their protocol is responsible for their bad to terrible outcomes. These outcomes can often be attributed to people selling products and family members who say they do not want patients to suffer by limiting their foods and drinks to their nutrigenomic diet requirements for optimal health.

Changing the way you eat in our Western society is a little bit like being at war. Everyone seems to be working against you. The media, the health food industry, and even your friends and family may question your choices and give you bad advice. They'll look to the popular media to understand what you are doing. For your sake and theirs, you'll need to be educated and know how to educate those around you about the WEE Protocol. It takes great resolve to follow the protocol for the long term, but it is worth all the effort to experience optimal health.

Over the last six years, I have used my unique nutrigenomic practice approach to help patients reverse symptoms, correct lab tests, and reverse terminal diseases. This approach works by removing toxic foods while replacing deficiencies with nutrient supplementation.

The following list summarizes the eight contributors to modern illness covered in the last section. The WEE Protocol works to correct, negate, or avoid these eight contributors. The section that follows the list provides more detail about how we do this with the WEE Protocol.

The eight contributors to modern illness are:

- We added genomically alien and plant-oil-based foods to our ancestral diet.
- We created metabolic confusion in our body's immune system by too much food variety.
- An omega-6 plant-oil-based diet caused excess cytokine stimulation without a natural omega-3 reserve for balance.
- We lost the minerals from our drinking water.
- We began consuming fruits and vegetables deficient in six essential nutrients.
- We developed increased latex sensitivities due to the marketing

of foods containing latex-like protein and our inhaling of latex fumes from tires on our roadways.

- Artificial chemicals, including monosodium glutamate (MSG) and artificial sweeteners, became prevalent in all processed foods.
- Microwaves created new chemical toxins in foods heated in plastics and sealed meal containers (simply microwaving food creates new chemicals).

The last two contributing factors on the list are perhaps the most straightforward to correct. Avoid processed foods that contain artificial chemicals, including monosodium glutamate (MSG), and avoid artificial sweeteners, even the ones labeled "natural." And avoid microwaving if at all possible.

Our general rule is that if a processed food has more than five ingredients, it is probably not something we should eat. This is not to say that if a food has less than five ingredients, it is fair game, or if it has more it is definitely out. Nevertheless, I've found this rule to be helpful in guiding patients through the grocery store.

Microwaves should be used minimally. Sometimes they are unavoidable, and in that case, food should be heated in the microwave in a glass container, not in a plastic one. Microwaves increase the rate at which plastics break down. When plastics break down, they release chemicals into our food, some of which may be harmful. Even plastics that are BPA free will break down and may release other toxic chemicals. Meals that are prepackaged and sealed in plastic should be avoided for the following reasons:

- they often contain artificial chemicals

- they are often heavily processed
- they usually require cooking in plastic in a microwave
- they have been in contact with plastic under variable conditions during storage

Diet and Supplements Work Together

The WEE Protocol uses supplements to correct the deficiencies in major nutrients, replace minerals lost from drinking water, and help balance omega-6 toxicity. The quantity of supplements required depends on the individual blood test results and how much the patient is willing to alter his or her diet.

For example, a patient who refuses to eliminate nuts, seeds, poultry, or other omega-6 foods will need to take more triple strength fish oil to achieve an omega-3 to omega-6 balance than a patient who has made the dietary changes.

Also, if the patient has the gluten sensitivity spectrum, as 95 percent of my patients do, and continue to consume gluten, then he or she will not absorb vitamins and minerals well and will require a larger quantity of supplements than a person with similar conditions who has eliminated gluten from his or her diet. Also, the gluten-related symptoms will not resolve.

For those suffering from gluten-related symptoms, no amount of supplements will resolve them. The only solution is to follow a gluten-free diet. However, just because an item is labeled gluten free doesn't mean you should eat it. Many popular gluten-free items in the marketplace are highly processed and high in omega-6 ingredients, such as nuts, seeds, teff, chia, flax, and soy. Also, while wheat is listed as one of the eight major allergens and clear labeling of wheat in food products is mandated by the FDA, gluten labeling is currently unregulated. A recent project of the American Dietetic Association documents that soy, millet, buckwheat, sorghum, and even white-rice flours test positive for high antigliadin.

Gluten-free labeling regulations have been proposed by the FDA, but as of July 2011, they have not been put into effect. The Gluten Intolerance Group (GIG) has a gluten-free certification program called the Gluten-Free Certification Organization (GFGO), which is a voluntary program to which manufacturers can submit. The GFCO is the only gluten-free certification process in the world. New science confirms that all oats contain avenin, a gluten-like compound.

Correcting Your Diet

Depending on your degree of latex sensitivity, you may need to avoid foods containing latex-like protein completely. Regardless of your level of sensitivity, the WEE Protocol recommends that all patients abstain from eating the following five foods: avocados, bananas, celery, figs, and kiwis. These foods have been found to always contain latex, and their negative impact on health outweighs any benefits of eating them.

The WEE Protocol also recommends that patients not eat fruits or vegetables picked out of season and artificially ripened. This includes out-of-season stone fruits, tomatoes, and peppers. Berries are generally all right to eat out of season, although they will taste better and cost less when purchased in season and then are

Nonhealing Wounds, Old Injuries, and Unresolved Pain
SHAUNA: MY "FORTIETH DOCTOR" PATIENT

My "Fortieth Doctor" patient was so named because I was the fortieth doctor she had seen for her nonhealing wound. She represents my uncovering, at that time, that there are latex-like proteins in at least thirteen fruits and vegetables. Although these proteins are undetectable to vision, taste, or smell, they had produced her profound latex chemical sensitivity disorder, which prevented her leg wound from healing for five years. Latex sensitive people react to eating foods laden with naturally occurring latex and latex-like proteins, such as avocados, bananas, celery, figs, kiwis, and out-of-season stone fruits. Recall from the section about Contributions to Modern Illness that picking fruits and vegetables in the green phase for better shipping results in the ongoing presence of the latex-like protein.

Shauna was a doctor in eastern Ohio where she had spent the last five years trying to heal a severe, open, draining wound on her own lower leg. The wound was six inches wide extending from her knee to her ankle. Unfortunately, she had failed to respond to any of the treatments prescribed over five years of referrals to thirty-nine other doctors and specialists in the Midwest and on the East Coast. This nonhealing wound from an automobile accident continued to embarrass this health care provider because she could not even heal her own wound. She came to me after a half a decade of failed traditional and nontraditional care, including surgeries, acupuncture, herbs, poultices, meditation, and yoga.

The biggest tip-off for me was that her wound always got worse when she had dental or gynecological care. Her wound flared whenever a dentist or doctor put gloved hands in her mouth or other openings for extended examinations or treatments.

Doing what's worked for the nearly five decades of my medical career, I spent the next few weeks doing medical literature searches to identify the likely culprit, in this case, the latex from the gynecologist's and dentist's gloves. Her response to latex gloves indicated that her doctors had not yet converted to the versions in use today that are almost latex free. I shared my research findings with her during her next visit, and her story became more interesting.

She told me that the wound flared when she ate certain foods. I determined that the trigger foods are those known to contain natural latex-like proteins, although she had not recognized the relationship. She confirmed that when she ate any of the thirteen

cont'd >

fruits and vegetables known to contain latex-like proteins naturally, she would not only flare but have near-syncope, passing
out episodes, presenting as weakness, fainting, or swooning.
She reported similar chemical sensitivity symptoms occurring,
although with less severity, when she entered rooms or build-
ings that had been recently painted with latex-based paints or
department store perfume or cosmetic areas.

After completely eliminating latex-laden foods, she began to
heal. On her next visit a few months later, the wound was completely healed, but she recounted trying a bit of banana a few
weeks before and had had to be treated by an EMS for anaphy-
laxis. This patient's decision to eat banana shows how easy it is
to discount health concerns even after you know how serious the
consequences can be, a pattern that can be lethal if you have a
terminal illness.

frozen for later, out-of-season use. Canned and frozen stone-fruits are low in latex since they are typically canned or frozen when ripe within the region they are grown.

Avoiding foods that are high in omega-6 fatty acids and low in omega-3 fatty acids is, for some, one of the most difficult dietary changes to make. Foods that should be eliminated to help balance the omega fatty acids include nuts, nut butters, and nut oils, seeds, seed butters, and seed oils, soy, soy derivatives, corn-fed poultry, farmed fish, corn oil, vegetable oil or shortening, margarine, chickpeas, and any foods containing these ingredients, including fried foods. Some people will find that after reaching optimal health, they can tolerate small amounts of these foods. These foods should not be tried until the monocyte percentage blood test, the marker the WEE Protocol uses for omega-6 toxicity, is around 5 percent or 3.5% in cancer patients.

By following the WEE Protocol recommendations for avoiding foods laden with latex-like protein and foods high in omega-6 and eliminating gluten, you will reduce the amount of genomically alien foods and decrease the variety of foods in your diet. Patients may find this simple eating difficult at first, especially if they are used to believing that the healthiest diets include exotic ingredients. A few weeks on a simple diet works wonders for new patients and families. It also saves money.

Part of relearning how to eat a healthful diet is understanding that there is much more to nutrigenomics than understanding "slow food" (the opposite of fast food), and the difference between foods grown organically and foods grown with pesticides, grass-fed beef versus grain-fed beef, eggs from free-range versus caged chickens, and so on. While most of these issues and concepts have great merit, for the last fifty years experts in these areas have totally missed the health concerns outlined in the WEE Protocol. We need to be vigilant in our food choices and careful from whom we accept our health advice.

The Influence of the USDA and Agribusiness

Another part of understanding where we are today with our food supply and eating habits is knowing the relationship between the modern United States Department of Agriculture (USDA) and agribusiness. Modern USDA and agribusiness research has at least two divisions. The first is science and research-based agribusiness, which is one of the foundation sources for new information about nutrigenomics.

The second is agribusiness as the business of selling food and health products, many of which are long known by the science and research-based division as less than healthy. For example, the science and research-based divisions understand that latex in foods, flax, and soy are unhealthful for many individuals. They also know how to produce cows, dairy products, eggs, goats, lambs, and pigs with higher levels of omega-3. Unfortunately, the agribusiness side does not choose to promote the most healthful food production methods (they are seen as less profitable), and we are left with the myriad of food issues I've described throughout this book.

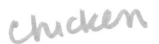

The way food is produced matters. The reason chicken and poultry are on the list of foods to avoid is because of the corn that chickens are fed. When a chicken eats corn, it stores the omega-6 fatty acids in its body. That is why chicken and poultry are very high in omega-6 fatty acids. If you had a chicken that was truly free-range and had not been fed corn, it would be a healthful food choice. However, it would also be a much leaner, smaller, and less profitable chicken. For this reason, it is very doubtful that you will find a chicken that has been produced without at least some corn being fed to it. Although solid science explains how to create health-giving poultry and poultry products, agribusiness continues to produce and market less than healthful poultry and poultry products.

Farmed fish have issues similar to those of poultry. Farm-raised salmon, for example, has significantly less omega-3 fatty acid and more omega-6 than its wild counterpart. In fact, eating farmed fish will only add to the levels of omega-6 in your body, whereas wild fish can help balance the omega-3 to omega-6 ratio by adding more omega-3 fatty acids. All farm-raised fish is less than healthful due to high omega-6 content from the corn it was fed. Farm-raised fish also pose health risks from higher levels of heavy metals from the farm field runoff.

Studies have shown that although there is some difference in the chemical composition between grass-fed and grain-fed beef, it is not appreciable in terms of omega-6 content. This is because cattle process grain differently than fish and poultry, and not all of it is stored in their bodies as omega-6. I do not differentiate

Chronic Fatigue, Fibromyalgia, and Insomnia
BETTY: MY "WHY DON'T DOCTORS GIVE A DAMN?" PATIENT

My "Why Don't Doctors Give a Damn?" patient's response to my greeting of "Hello, I am Dr. Aukerman. What can I do to help?" made me do a double take, asking, "What?"

Betty explained she had been to countless primary care doctors and specialists, but it seemed to her that doctors didn't seem to care about their patients anymore. She reasoned this from her observation that when the doctor's treatment solution was of no value, the doctor would say, "You did not respond to the treatment," as if it was the patient's choice not to respond. I was curious about how she expressed her thought process, so I kept going on this topic.

"So, what are you looking for in your ideal doctor?" I asked. She said simply, "Doctors used to care enough to find out what was really the cause of your problems and not simply give up when the prescription did nothing and blame the patient for not responding."

As it turns out, this patient had been suffering from severe fibromyalgia, chronic fatigue, and a sleep disorder for at least a decade—little wonder she felt betrayed by the entire medical profession. By the completion of the visit, she had managed to get me to commit to researching her conditions in "PubMed.gov" and promising a solution for her next visit in a month or so.

On my way home from the clinic that evening, I realized what it was about her story that got to me; it was my story too. Until that moment on the way home, I had nearly forgotten that I had quit practicing about a decade earlier, after twenty-six-and-a-half years of practice, partially due to fibromyalgia, chronic fatigue, and my sleep disorder. I had compartmentalized it until this patient focused me on her and thereby on myself.

Responding to this renewed insight, I stopped at the pharmacy to get my own supplies to begin developing what was eventually to become an extremely successful treatment for fibromyalgia, chronic fatigue, and sleep disorders. You see, at the end of her visit, I had suggested she combine several program elements with which I had found individual successes, timed-release vitamin B complex for her problem of getting to sleep, magnesium oxide and calcium carbonate for her trouble staying asleep and to reduce fibromyalgia pain, and high-potency omega-3 fish oil to compensate for the excess plant oils in her diet that increased her pain, ruined her sleep, and made her grumpy. Additionally, I asked her to avoid the thirteen foods containing latex-like protein to reduce her fibromyalgia symptoms since they magnify pain by eight to ten times.

Starting that evening, I, too, began to take my newly created treatment program with the four components that I had recommended with some success for other patients with similar symptom sets.

cont'd >

Because I had committed to the patient to develop a successful program for her fibromyalgia, chronic fatigue, and sleep disorder, I needed to start the same program so I could relieve my own symptoms. I also had to know if any part of the program did not work before she came back for her next visit.

I was concerned when I was not improved at the end of the first week, so I increased the dose to the next level. I continued to increase the dose each week until, by the fifth week, all my fibromyalgia symptoms of 17.5 years had disappeared completely. To my continued pleasure, my fibromyalgia has not returned over the last five years since I continued at the same dose as the fifth week. In addition, my chronic fatigue was 80 percent gone by the fifth week. The sleeplessness improved by 50 percent by the fifth

between grass-fed beef or lamb and grain-fed beef or lamb when recommending them to my meat-eating patients.

Learn the Rules of Coming Back to the Basics

The principles of the WEE Protocol are, at the core, very basic and revolve around the concept of eating and living simply. The heart week. My symptoms have continued to improve for the last five years to the negligible level they are today.

When my patient returned for her six-week appointment, she reported a 50 percent improvement of each of her symptoms for the first time in a decade. I reported to her the next step she could try since she was seeking greater relief than she had achieved. When she returned at twelve weeks, she reported complete relief from the fibromyalgia, chronic fatigue, and sleep disorder when she followed the program completely, and an 80 percent improvement if she missed doses or ate the latex-containing foods. She was satisfied with a physician for the first time in a decade, thanks to the effort we made together to resolve her problems.

of the WEE Protocol can be summarized by six nutrigenomic rules of reasonableness. When you learn about the seemingly radical changes needed to bring your health back to optimal, the dos and don'ts can seem daunting. By learning the rules of reasonableness, you can use them as a guide as you work through the protocol.

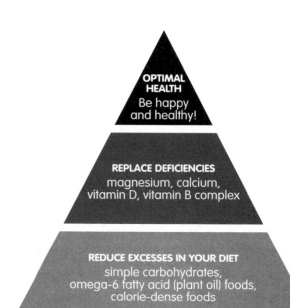

The Pyramid to Better Health through Nutrigenomics

Figure 4. *The nutrigenomic pyramid emphasizes removing toxic foods and compounds and reducing excesses in the diet so that we can use fewer expensive supplements to regain health.*

Nutrigenomic Rules of Reasonableness

- What you eat always controls the impact of your genes on your body.
- Limit the variety of your foods to ancestral foods.
- Reduce excesses and replenish deficiencies through supplementation and diet changes.

- Avoid products and advice based solely on research conducted on rats.
- Avoid health advice from people who cannot guide you to achieve perfect lab results.
- Make sure your life has a balance of work and rest.

The Health-Care Provider's Role in the WEE Protocol

For the health-care provider's part of the WEE Protocol, we work to define your problems accurately or identify the problem's metabolic cause precisely enough to account for each symptom, abnormal lab marker, and disease. Correct definition of the problem enables patients to bring about significant improvements and, potentially, a cure through natural means.

We also perceive the underlying principal nutritional pathways that produce symptoms, abnormal lab markers, and disease processes. Once these are identified, we can identify the processes needed to advance down the road toward optimal health.

Most modern Western doctors appear to be unaware of the nutritional, physiologic, or situational causes for the symptoms, the associated lab test results, and diseases of their patients. Their records would support that they were unaware of the underlying nutritional basis for their patient's diseases and conditions at the time of their last visit, before their patients came to my practice looking for answers. The doctors also were not responding to the desperate frustration expressed by their patients looking for answers.

Over these six years and more than 32,000 patient visits, while reaching out to the many patients who were desperately trying to turn their health around, I recognized and compiled a number of points that they failed to grasp before coming to their first nutrigenomic lecture. I require all new patients and families to attend an introductory nutrigenomics lecture. I also strongly suggest that they attend the multiple, optional WEE Protocol education classes. Unfortunately, their doctors and/or other health advisors did not appear to have sufficient nutritional knowledge to prevent their patients from falling into an abyss of disease and dis-ease. Until now, no one source brought all this critical information together.

As I uncovered these nutrigenomic pathways leading to illness and those leading back to optimal health, I then worked through the new information with the patients and their families so they could make the nutritional changes needed. My patients appeared to "magically" lose symptoms, and their once abnormal lab tests resolved to normal. Better yet, their lab tests went to the optimal range. The optimal range is the term I use for labs in the best range to restore health, which is the upper ninetieth percentile of accepted reference ranges for tests such as for magnesium, calcium, and Vitamin D, and the lower twelfth percent for tests such as for parathyroid hormone (PTH). Within weeks to months, their diseases lightened and eventually were not detectable in the clinical or lab setting.

The foundation of the WEE Protocol, as illustrated in Figure 4, is removing toxic foods. All patients should avoid latex and latex-like proteins in foods. Although not every patient has classic celiac disease or gluten sensitivity, about ninety-five percent of my patients do have a significant gluten sensitivity that requires the reduction or elimination of gluten from the diet. Gluten sensitivities including celiac disease do not always manifest as gastrointestinal problems and can therefore go unrecognized by the patient. I use a variety of factors, including blood work, to diagnose gluten sensitivity. Some patients with celiac disease or gluten sensitivity also do not tolerate gluten-like substitutes. These substitutes include xanthan and guar gums, maltodextrin, and modified food starch. Oats, soy, buckwheat, millet, and sorghum also have gluten-like compounds only recently recognized when using very sensitive ELISA antigliadin testing. Additionally, research has show that avenin, a protein found in oats, can cause bowel damage similar to that produced by gluten in people with celiac disease. This is why some people with celiac disease do not tolerate oats. Research has shown that prolamins in various foods cross react and do the same.

Although we are deficient in many vitamins and minerals, our diet contains many excesses. Most people in America eat too many calories, too many simple carbohydrates, and too much omega-6 fatty acid. By reducing these excesses and bringing our carbohydrate, calorie, and omega-6 fatty acid intake into balance, we can reverse the toxicities created by these excesses.

Loren Cordain et al. in the landmark article on "The Origins and Evolution of the Western Diet, Health Implications for the Twenty-First Century," documented the massive changes in our macronutrients over the last 10,000 years, but the most drastic changes happened in the last twenty-five to fifty years. The article noted that in the Western diet, people consume:

- twenty to thirty times the normal amount of omega-6 plant oil from seeds (including flax), nuts, poultry, avocados, etc.
- 200 percent excess in refined carbohydrates (mostly gluten-based), leading to the devastating celiac epidemic
- 100 percent excess proteins and salt, leading to the U.S. domination in renal failure cases

Cancer

LISA: MY "I JUST WANT TO LIVE LONG ENOUGH TO SEE MY CHILD INTO GRADE SCHOOL" PATIENT, ALSO KNOWN AS "THE PATIENT THAT STARTED IT ALL"

You were introduced to this patient earlier in the book. Now I'll share the whole story. My "I Just Want to Live Long Enough to See My Child into Grade School" patient had taken a year out of chemotherapy for breast cancer to have a baby. Soon after delivery, Lisa was told she had moved to stage IV cancer and had sixty days to live. Being the consummate mother, she came to our center with an unusual request: "I just want to live long enough to see my child get into grade school."

After our tears had cleared, I made a commitment to her and myself to devote my spare time in research mode to see if I could identify something new that was not already being done by her competent specialists. I was searching for something else she could do to increase her chance of surviving for the time needed to see her baby enter grade school. After all, she had one of the best cancer doctors in the area if not in the country, so it was not likely that I could add much on that level. Therefore, I devoted my research to finding those nutritional elements that favor cancer survival and those that favor the prevention of cancers.

As providence would have it, about six weeks into her sixty days to live and into my research efforts, I uncovered a peer-reviewed nutrition journal article entitled "Preventing Cancer with the Use of Long Chain Omega-3 Fatty Acids" or fish oil. At 3:30 in the morning,

I read the authors' work, which shared algorithms (flowcharts) and grids (tables) outlining many cell-stimulating cytokines. The research provided me with a potential road map to how cancers develop from the omega-6 plant oil in our foods. It also showed no cancers developing from the omega-3 oils (DHA/EPA) in our food.

I set about researching each of the cytokines listed on the grid to sort out the breast cancer cytokines. Unfortunately, breast cancer comes from each of the omega-6 cytokine chains, meaning she and I would have to approach the whole grid at once, a full field attack on all sites for cancer.

The next morning, I called my patient into the office to see if she was still interested in anything that might help. She was so excited and grateful for any hope, any possibility for survival, that she came after she got off work, and we began our journey of discovery that would last the next three years.

The article I found that morning referred me to a free software program called KIM-2, or Keep It Managed, available from the NIH Web site, efaeducation.nih.gov. The program helped identify foods that might improve my patient's chances and also identified foods that could have been making the cancer grow aggressively. The foods that were causing harm included seeds, nuts, avocados, hummus, poultry, flax, soy, and many more.

The authors suggested in their article that remission from breast cancer was possible if a patient lowered the ratio of omega-6 plant oil foods to no more than 2.5 times the level of the omega-3

cont'd >

foods in the diet (compared to the western diet of twenty to thirty times). Furthermore, the authors of the article postulated that a man with prostate cancer needed to lower the ratio of omega-6 plant oil foods to no more than 2.2 times the omega-3 foods in his diet for a remission of cancer. The authors also postulated that if a person had lung cancer, he or she would need to lower the level of omega-6 foods to 2 times the omega-3 foods in his or her diet. I now ask every patient to use KIM-2 since we uncovered it for this deserving mother. And we now teach a weekly class on KIM-2.

My patient's diet contained a great deal of seeds, nuts, avocados, hummus, poultry, and other foods expected to make the cancer grow per the KIM-2 program. We modified her diet by adding foods quieting to her immune system, reaching a 2.5:1 ratio, which corresponds to a monocyte count of less than 6 percent. Relating the ratio to the monocyte count is done using a formula I developed from other articles using the monocyte percentage as a proxy for omega-6 plant oil.

Thanks to Lisa, I now had two tools: the KIM-2 program and the monocyte percentage from the CBC, which let me know where I am in quieting down the plant oil stimulation for the growth of cancer in humans. In time, I would discover that these tools are useful in treating every symptom and condition for most modern diseases since plant-oil excess figures in their correction.

Immediately, we set out with our new program. Even though she had continued to receive chemo, her cancer marker was very high and climbing. Within the last month of what had been her original life expectancy estimate, as we lowered her monocyte percentage, she began to lower her cancer marker. As a good story goes, in six months, her cancer doctor pronounced her in remission and even stopped her chemo.

I kept working with my patient because remissions do not always last. Her cancer doctors were especially confident about the remission, so they stopped her chemotherapy.

Unfortunately, after about 16 months of remission, I noted the cancer marker that had been flat was now starting to climb. Immediately, I e-mailed her cancer doctor who was surprised that I had cared enough to follow her. Surprised that her cancer markers were rising, he decided she was no longer in a remission.

When I started working with this patient, the center had hired a practice manager/coordinator who was an art therapist. Because she had a counseling background, I asked her to assist me in conducting classes and one-on-one teaching of the programming I had developed for the WEE Protocol for applied nutrigenomics.

By the time this patient was out of remission, our team was becoming an outstanding asset. By attending my lectures as I taught patients and families, a team approach was developed for explaining the body of my work. The counseling background of team members gave us insights into how difficult it is for patients and families to change old ideas about foods now known to be unhealthful.

The life and journey of my patient became more complicated once she had a recurrence; her cancer doctors wanted her in a clinical trial that they felt precluded participating in our nutrition programs.

cont'd >

She died about sixteen weeks after quitting our protocol, giving me my first notice that I needed to do special teaching to patients and families on how to protect themselves from others who may mean well but use old information that will not help them. Rather, it harms them. The table shows this patient's progress, both before, during, and after following the WEE Protocol.

I discovered that patients do not survive very long—usually from six to sixteen weeks—once they end our protocol if they are terminal. I now believe the WEE Protocol diet could have protected this patient and others, but they would have to learn to live the diet completely. This provides me with evidence, if not proof, that the WEE Protocol I had developed is not a cure but a very successful treatment adjunct for cancers if patients and families attend the classes, ask the right questions, take the correct nutrients, and eat the correct foods and stay on traditional therapy (chemo, radiation, surgery).

As I would later understand more clearly, it is a very successful treatment adjunct for nearly all diseases known to humans or, at the very least, to all diseases we have researched to the date of this writing, some 250 and counting.

About two years after I developed the WEE Protocol, the CEO of a prestigious cancer center, his deputy, and several leading cancer center doctors requested a meeting with me at the Center for Integrative Medicine. Expecting them to request that I cease all treatment of their patients because they believed I was contaminating their research trials, I asked the office manager to attend to be sure we clearly heard their message. I asked my usual opening at meetings without a known agenda: "So, what can I do for you?" I expected a very negative or nonsupportive retort, since, up until this time, there had been no contact or communication, unofficial or official, by anyone from the medical center. I was greatly surprised by their response!

The renowned CEO cancer physician said, "Our nurses, patient care resource managers (PCRMS), doctors, oncology techs, our patients, and their families have been reporting that our patients feel better, are happy and always in a good mood, do not get sick with chemo, do not lose their hair with chemo, and appear to be doing better if they are on your program."

I asked, "What do you mean by, 'They seem to be doing better'?"

The CEO responded, "They seem to be not dying."

I laughed out loud and asked again, "What can I do for you?"

The CEO asked if I would be comfortable if they did research over my shoulder as I worked with stage IV cancer patients to see why, how, and if I was really achieving any of these five miracles.

Amazed and happy, I agreed to proceed. Since then, I have done a great deal of work with cancer patients and their families at this Big-10 university and major cancer center in the United States. It continues to amaze me how these seemingly insignificant changes can have such a huge impact in the health and quality of life of so many.

The Progress of Cancer Patient Lisa

Date	Breast Carcinoma Antigen CA27.29)	Date	Breast Carcinoma Antigen CA27.29)
beginning of diagnosis		24 Aug 2006	426.0
10 Oct 2004	1276.0	16 Dec 2006	355.0
07 Nov 2004	1266.0	told cancer in remission	
04 Dec 2004	960.0	27 Jan 2007	424.0
original response to her chemotherapy		10 Feb 2007	420.0
		17 May 2007	924.0
03 Jan 2005	694.0	I called the oncologist surgeon who restarted chemo but stopped the Wee Protocol program	
05 Feb 2005	734.0		
28 Apr 2005	901.0		
23 Jun 2005	1058.0	09 Aug 2007	2679.0
20 Jul 2005	1288.0	08 Nov 2007	7733.0
First saw the patient		29 Nov 2007	7602.0
18 Aug 2005	1293.0	21 Dec 2007	5594.0
15 Sept 2005	1618.0	11 Jan 2008	5053.0
Wee Protocol started		01 Feb 2008	5405.0
13 Oct 2005	1755.0	22 Feb 2008	5536.0
17 Nov 2005	2042.0	20 Mar 2008	5560.0
WEE Protocol starting to work		17 Apr 2008	11637.0
14 Dec 2005	1838.0	15 May 2008	8851.0
11 Feb 2006	1005.0	28 Jun 2008	13311.0
09 Mar 2006	745.0	02 Jul 2008	17106.0
06 Apr 2006	507.0	23 Jul 2008	20106.0
01 Jun 2006	422.0	death	

Supplements

Part of the WEE Protocol involves using corrective elements, or supplements, to help correct deficiencies and balance toxicities. What supplements and the corrective dosages are needed is determined by review of the patient's WEE Protocol 90/360 Lab Assessment. The assessment includes the following tests:

- **Complete blood count (CBC) and differential:** This test's differential is used for determining the monocyte percentage, which is the lab marker we use to determine the level of omega-6 toxicity. This tells us if the patient has been exposed to too much omega-6 plant oil and in our over 32,000 patient-visit experience if it is over 5 percent, the condition may be disease producing.

- **Calcium, magnesium, vitamin D, and intact parathyroid hormone (PTH):** These tests enable us to determine the level of mineral reserves in bones and how much bone PTH is removing to influence your energy level and regulates total cholesterol and LDL levels.

- **C-reactive protein:** This test is our proxy for the acute phase reactant (APR) level in the body. APR levels indicate systemic inflammation. C-reactive protein levels are also used as a marker for cardiac health.

- **Lipids:** We use your lipid profile (HDL) as a proxy for vitamin B2 and the total cholesterol and LDL as proxy for your calcium, magnesium, and vitamin D levels.

- **Thyroid-stimulating hormone (TSH) and thyroxine-related tests (T4, T3, and uptakes):** These tests show us how your

Eating Disorders

SAM: MY "I'M HAVING TROUBLE WITH COMPLIANCE" PATIENT

Sam, a forty-six-year-old marketing research engineer, has metabolic syndrome without a terminal disease but with all typical metabolism-related diagnoses: abnormal lipids, gout, hypertension, hypothyroidism, multiple nighttime urinations, obesity, sleep apnea, and a history of kidney stones. These diagnoses point to his adult celiac disease genes actively creating problems.

After the WEE Protocol Intake and Assessment, I suggested to Sam that he try these nutrients to balance deficiencies and excesses in his diet:

- calcium carbonate and magnesium oxide plus additional vitamin D3
- balanced time-released vitamin B complex (without vitamin C)
- cinnamon bark without extract or chromium
- triple strength fish oil with 900 milligrams of EPA/DHA per 1,360/1,400 milligram capsule
- multivitamin for age and gender with lutein and lycopene

These nutrients are usually best taken before meals and at bedtime. Any missed daytime doses can be taken if the patient gets up at night after 2:00 A.M. for any reason, such as nighttime urination.

Sam provided a wonderful example of a person who, despite every lab abnormality and disease label related to metabolic disease, coupled with a lifetime of an eating disorder, was still able to pull off remarkable improvements. All he achieved is a testimony to what the WEE Protocol is able to do, despite Sam's very complex lifestyle and despite sometimes falling off the treatment protocol largely as a result of his eating disorder and bipolar and ADD issues. Nonetheless, Sam deserves all the credit for his changes!

Sam's eating disorder and his bipolar and ADD issues each contributed to his need for extra compliance, classes, and most likely more nutrients than most patients would require because of his reduced food compliance.

The root cause of Sam's metabolic syndrome was his adult celiac genes, which effectively blocked his uptake of calcium, magnesium, vitamins A, B, B12, D, E, K, and caused a great deal of his lactose intolerance. Once his antigliadin antibodies fall below 1.0 and stay there uninterrupted for at least nine months, Sam would be able to eat about 10 percent of the prior gluten and need little supplementation, a bonus for compliance since supplements cost, food choices do not.

Sam's poor gluten compliance was reflected in the fact that his calcium, magnesium, and vitamin D levels did not quickly move to their 90 percent levels of 9.9 for calcium, 2.5 for magnesium, and 90 for vitamin D. He also had high antigliadin IGG, which documents significant bowel damage. He also had high levels of

cont'd >

the IGA, which documents immune disease generation capacity and his current exposure to glutens.

Sam, so far, has been able to walk away from type 2 diabetes, defined as HgbA1c greater than 6.1, by implementing mild carbohydrate changes and by his terrific response to cal-mag-D and cinnamon supplements.

In summary, Sam has everything in the metabolic syndrome basket with his extra bipolar and ADD issues. After working the WEE Protocol together, we were able to achieve the following results:

- Metabolic syndrome related diagnoses are gone or improving. None have gotten worse even with poor compliance.

thyroid is functioning and can point to gluten sensitivity if your TSH is above 1.0.

- **Thyroid antibody tests (TPO), antigliadin antibodies (IGG, IGA), and celiac genes (HLA DQ 2, 8):** These tests point to gluten effects on the thyroid, pituitary, bowel, and immune system. The celiac gene test can be helpful in pointing toward gluten issues, but not having the gene doesn't preclude you from celiac autoimmune consequences or gluten sensitivity.
- There is no useful traditional lab test for latex-like protein effects on the body, although the Westergren Sedimentation

- Abnormal lipids have improved, even with poor compliance.
- Gout is gone.
- Sleep apnea is improving.
- Frequency of getting up at night to urinate, down from six times per night to two times per night, even with poor compliance.
- Hypothyroidism is improving, but gluten compliance issues remain.
- Hypertension is gone and those medications have been stopped.
- Obesity has improved slightly with twenty-three pounds of weight loss even with very poor compliance.

Rate, ANA (antinuclear antibody), and C-reactive protein are most likely impacted and elevated by the presence of ingested latex-like proteins. Clinical signs are red chin, cheeks, ears, and latex lines on neck and upper chest.

After considerable research, I formulated a replacement program for deficits in the B vitamins, calcium, magnesium, vitamin D, and trace minerals by adding together multivitamins, balanced time-released vitamin B complex, and calcium carbonate, magnesium oxide, and

Two Stories of Relapsing Multiple Sclerosis
ANNA AND ROSE: MY "DISEASE VANISHED, SPECIALIST THINKS HE DIAGNOSED ME WRONG" PATIENTS

Two unrelated female patients in their forties and fifties came to me after receiving diagnoses of relapsing multiple sclerosis (MS). They saw different MS specialists in different cities, but shared a remarkably similar story.

Both specialists made the diagnoses in January and recon-firmed the diagnoses at June follow-up visits. These ladies, unknown to each other, had both come to one of my community education classes on nutrigenomic nutrition in June. They each came to see me for an office appointment afterward. They each related that they were originally frightened by the hopelessness of their diagnosis: relapsing multiple sclerosis, not drug treatable. This was made more serious and devastating to them because their neurologists were nationally recognized leaders in the field. Both patients were told by these specialists that no available effec-tive treatment existed for them.

Both patients recounted to me that they left the nutrigenomic class knowing they must never eat gluten again. Both were seen, evaluated, and started on my WEE Protocol for MS the same week in mid-June. Per their protocols, their nutrients were adjusted based on their original lab set drawn about a week or so after their original visit, then readjusted at the six- to eight-week reassessment visit based on the six- to eight-week lab results, their symptoms, and their clinical appearances. This is the way the protocol is designed.

So far this does not sound too amazing, but what follows made time stop for each of these ladies and for me. When these ladies went to see their MS specialists, both neurologists and leaders in the MS field, in September in two different cities, one-hundred miles apart, their resulting visits were recounted identically. Both neurologists were reported to have told their patients, "I must have been mistaken the last two visits in diagnosing you as relapsing MS since your symptoms are all gone, your head CT scans are resolved, and you appear to be well neurologically. My patients with relapsing MS do not get well without drug treatment, and you have had no drug treatment. As a specialist, I have no other explanation other than that the wrong diagnosis was made."

We physicians have such faith in our training, our testing, and our past experiences that we do not recognize them as real when such amazing things happen to our patients. Traditionally, we recant them as errors rather than attempt to replicate the patient's success by improvising on current treatment protocols.

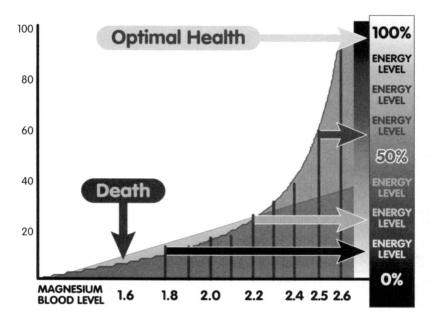

Figure 5 caption: Magnesium levels are critical for maintaining energy levels and reaching optimal health.

vitamin D. I added fish oil supplements to counter omega-6 excesses and cinnamon bark to help protect against carbohydrate excesses.

These supplements work to improve the lab test results as follows:

- Centrum Silver multivitamin or the equivalent for nonmenstruating patients or Centrum regular or the equivalent for those who menstruate provides the Recommended Dietary Allowance (RDA) of trace minerals and vitamins A and E. Multivitamins should include lutein and lycopene but should be free of added herbs or plant materials to avoid latex.

- Balanced vitamin B complex timed-release supplements, referred to on some labels as B-100TR or B-50TR, are used to increase good cholesterol (HDL) to greater than 60. It also lowers C-reactive protein. Our ideal level of C-reactive protein is zero. The balanced, time-released B-complex supplements also will calm restless leg syndrome and produce melatonin to get you to sleep if taken early in the day but stopped before 5:00 p.m. (or earlier for some patients, depending on dose).
- Calcium carbonate, magnesium oxide, and vitamin D supplements, often purchased all in one and referred to as cal-mag-D, are used to increase levels of all three in the blood but do not have adequate Vitamin D. It is also used to lower intact parathyroid hormone (PTH) to less than fourteen. Today, we start with a cal-mag-D product (rather than separate calcium and magnesium) for better bowel tolerance and support.
  - Calcium carbonate is dosed to produce blood calcium levels in the upper level of the reference range, usually greater than 9.8. Calcium at this level will do amazing things for the muscles and joints.
  - Magnesium oxide is dosed to produce blood magnesium levels in the upper reference range, usually greater than 2.5. It will do amazing things for bones, bowels, and brains. As the magnesium level increases, the patient's energy level also increases, as show in Figure 5.
  - Vitamin D3 is dosed to reach the upper 10 percent of the reference range. Usually this requires an additional vitamin D supplement.

- Triple strength fish oil is used to balance omega-6 toxicity. We use monocyte blood cell counts to track omega-6 toxicity. When your monocyte percentage is less than five, which is written in blood work results as <5, and your red blood cell distribution width (RDW) is less than 15 (<15) and you have normal platelets, we consider your omega-3 and omega-6 intake balanced. Omega-3 fish oil decreases inflammation and related conditions only if the content of EPA and DHA is greater than 50 percent per weight in each capsule or teaspoonful. The best supplements contain 70 percent or more of EPA and DHA and are referred to by some manufacturers as triple strength fish oil and has 900 mg or greater of EPA and DHA per capsule.
- Cinnamon bark (without chromium or extract) is helpful for reducing triglycerides. Our goal for triglycerides is less than 70 (<70). Cinnamon bark supplements also lower HgbA1c to less than 5.0 (<5.0) unless diabetes has become fixed.

Choose Foods Free of Latex-like Proteins

As described previously, latex-like proteins are toxins created naturally by fruits and vegetables. They store their carbohydrates (i.e., sugars and starches) and proteins as a bitter compound while they are in the green stage of growth and development. This is an ecologically occurring defense which happens presumably to deter animals from eating the fruit or vegetable before it is mature and ready to spread its seeds. In nature, this latex-like protein is converted back to sugar, starch, and protein when the food is naturally ripened on the vine, plant, or tree by the plant hormone ethylene. This conversion process does not occur if the fruits and vegetables are picked while green and artificially ripened using synthetic/artificial ethylene gas, called banana gas or welder's gas. Instead, the latex-like protein remains intact. It subsequently causes injury when eaten by those sensitized by inhaling auto tire fumes and latex products such as IV tubing and gloves containing latex.

Of the original thirteen foods listed, five of them, avocados, bananas, celery, figs, and kiwis, whether in nature or in the food delivery chain, never ripen their latex-like protein back to simple protein and carbohydrates. They always retain a latex-like protein, which enhances allergies and chemical sensitivities and suppresses the human immune system's resistance to diseases, such as infections, and permits cancer growth during the time it suppresses the immune system. Any food that is picked in the "green" growth phase, that is, unripened, will have latex-like proteins. This includes health products containing unripened wheat grass, barley grass, or supplements with live components extracted from fruits and vegetables that were not completely tree, vine, or plant ripened.

According to scientists, totally ripened fruit is found only on the ground since it is the ethylene hormone that in nature deactivates the latex, which holds the fruit to the bush, tree, or vine. Similarly, out-of-season vegetables contain latex-like protein when still unripened by the plant. When they are artificially ripened, the latex-like protein persists. An example of artificially ripened produce is found in the tomatoes available in the grocery during the winter. These out-of-season, out-of-region foods are, in contrast, picked green enough to withstand being transported in a cargo ship for months at sea. Higher concentrations of latex-like proteins are found in them as a result, especially if they have a green stem attached. Because canned and frozen fruits and vegetables are processed close to the area where they are grown, they are picked closer to the ripened stage and have less latex-like proteins.

The latex-like protein is not present in leaf vegetables such as kale, lettuce, and spinach, or in the flower stalks or bloom components of plants such as asparagus, broccoli, Brussels sprouts, cabbage, and cauliflower. In other words, regardless of the season or when they were picked, these are not laden with latex. Latex in tomatoes, potatoes, and green peppers convert with cooking.

We teach our patients that these five foods (banana, avocado, celery, kiwi, and fig) often promote the diseases from which they suffer and do not offer any health benefits in today's abundant food supply. We recommend that all of our patients avoid these five foods. Out-of-season, artificially ripened stone fruits are also not recommended. Canned stone fruits are expected to be free of latex-like protein. Today, many more fruits, vegetables, and products made from artificially ripened fruits and vegetables have been identified as containing latex-like proteins that deteriorate our health and, yes, can even stimulate growth in and promote our next cancer or degenerative disease. Eating latex-laden foods impairs the immune system.

FOR EXTRA RESEARCH: Search for key words and phrases such as "latex-like proteins in food" or "latex fruit syndrome" in your internet browser and on PubMed.gov.

We recommend that patients avoid latex-like proteins in processed food and health-food products by avoiding products labeled as containing "live" or "alive" ingredients from the five foods or their components that we know to contain latex-like proteins. The terms "live" and "alive" on these products are often marketing ploys, and the products in those vitamins and supplements are no more alive than those that are often accused of being inorganic.

While there is nothing wrong with raw foods, and probiotics can be good for your gut, these heavily processed and marketed products often contain harmful components of foods that are high in latex-like proteins and omega-6 fatty acids.

Educate your health professionals or seek those who appear to be educable about the latex-like protein toxicity in foods so you are not struggling alone to reach better health.

Fibromyalgia may be best understood when viewed as arrested healing. Healing occurs when any or all of the following are in effect:

- An absence of latex-like protein in foods that flare inflammation and magnify pain, such as avocados, bananas, celery, figs, and kiwis. There are eight stone fruits and vegetables that may be latex free if they are truly tree, vine, or plant ripened, which allows conversion of the latex back to sugar and protein. Avocados, bananas, celery, figs, and kiwis never convert their latex.

- An omega-3:omega-6 ratio of 1:1, or very close to it, which translates into having a monocyte count (i.e., as shown in the CBC with differential) at or close to 3.5 percent. This can be produced with omega-3 fish oil as a pain/inflammation reducer, and with the reduction of omega-6 plant oil in foods.
- A cal-mag-D product for better bowel tolerance and support, with effectiveness of mineral replacement monitored by testing to get the intact PTH<14.
- Calcium carbonate supplements that produce blood calcium levels in the upper level of the reference range, usually greater than 9.8. Such levels will do amazing things for the muscles and joints.
- Magnesium oxide supplements that produce blood magnesium levels in the upper reference range, usually greater than 2.5, which will do amazing things for bones, bowels, and brains.

Chronic fatigue and sleep disorders are best understood when viewed as the nervous system being dysfunctional, irritated, agitated, and uncomfortable when certain vitamins or minerals are not in perfect balance. Sleep disorder is best understood as occurring when our normal sleep function is disturbed by anything that interferes with melatonin production or its effectiveness in the brain which occurs in the passages of soft tissues that swell when B-complex is deficient. For these problems, we recommend:

- **Calcium carbonate:** Supplements that produce blood calcium in the upper level of the reference range, usually greater than 9.8, will do amazing things to quiet the nerves and tissues and relax the muscles.
- **Magnesium oxide:** Supplements that produce blood magnesium levels in the upper reference range, usually greater than 2.5, will do amazing things to quiet restless legs and nerves.
- **Vitamin B:** A balanced vitamin B complex formulated to release over a long time span will calm restless leg syndrome, produce melatonin, and support sleep if taken before 5:00 P.M. as well as reducing snoring and gingivitis.
- Increased diurnal sunlight exposure helps makes melatonin to promote sleep but only with adequate time-released Vitamin B complex. Wear sunglasses for driving to protect the eyes, but they are not necessary at all times when you are outdoors, and if used continually, sunglasses will increase insomnia by breaking the melatonin production cycle.

The Importance of Staying on the WEE Protocol

Our first patient died in a recurrence approximately sixteen months after being taken off the program. The progress of her cancer before, during, and after participating in the WEE Protocol is documented in the table on page 76. The shift in her progress made us aware of the need to teach the basics plus self-protection skills.

Our second cancer patient died from the complications of surgery for intracranial metastasis while on the WEE Protocol. Her cancer was controlled when she died, showing we had been effective in teaching these new principles about self-protection to the second patient. We learned the following from these experiences:

- We need to teach patients and families to protect themselves from others who often mean well but come with fears or old information that will set patients back in their progress.
- Patients will not survive long off our program if they are terminal unless they have really learned the diet in our program, continue to live it, and change their disease producing chemistry.
- I had developed an effective evidence-based treatment adjunct for cancer, not a cure.
- I had developed an effective evidence-based treatment for all diseases that we researched, not a cure.

The science behind this lesson is complex, with several variables to consider:

- Omega-6 plant oil stimulates cancer growth and metastasis.
- Omega-3 fish oil (EPA/DHA) quiets cancer growth, prevents or slows metastasis, and with time-release Vitamin B complex and magnesium lowers the C-reactive protein, an acute phase reactant, for better chemotherapy effects.
- Latex-like proteins in foods suppress the immune protection against cancer and favor cancer growth for forty-eight hours after those foods are consumed.
- Timed-release vitamin B complex supplements prevent or reverse neuropathy and hair loss from chemotherapy agents and lower the C-reactive protein, an acute phase reactant.
- Calcium-magnesium-Vitamin D (cal-mag-D) supplements enhance the body's protection against ovarian, prostate, and

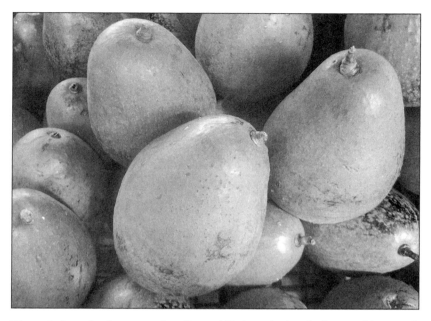

Figure 6. *Avocados, bananas, celery, figs, and kiwis are foods we're forever told are good for us, but they can be extremely damaging to our health.* SOURCE: *wikimediacommons.org,* Copyright 2005 David Monniaux

gastrointestinal cancers, and lowers C-reactive protein, an acute phase reactant, for best chemotherapy effect.

- Cinnamon slows sugar-simulated cancer growth from carbohydrates in meals and is now slowly being recognized as an anti-cancer herb.

FOR EXTRA RESEARCH: Use your Internet browser to search for the term, "KIM-2, NIH" to better understand the content of omega-6 fatty acids in your food supply. These fatty acids lead to the modern disease epidemics. Knowing how to avoid them will protect you and your family.

Metabolic Diseases: All Diseases Are Metabolic

The WEE Protocol is effective at correcting metabolic eating disorders, which include lipid disorders (i.e., elevated cholesterol, triglycerides, and LDL, or low HDL), metabolic syndromes (i.e., fatty liver, gout, hypertension, obesity, polycystic ovarian syndrome, and type 2 diabetes), and eating disorders (i.e., binging, bulimia, cravings, gastroparesis, and habituations).

Using metabolic eating disorders as an example, the diagnosis of a specific eating disorder does not adequately describe the scope of the patient's problem. Our patient Sam in the case study, at forty-five years of age, was ill before the diagnosis of the metabolic eating disorder was made. People are often ill for months and years before a metabolic eating disorder is known or suspected. Even after the diagnosis of hypertension, lipids, and obesity, Sam was still very ill because making the diagnoses does not correct any of the abnormal metabolism or chemistry behind the disease.

Bariatric surgery is important for those with terminal metabolic eating disorders, but even when surgery is successful, it simply removes one source of the disease focus, the physical site for food absorption. Often it temporarily fixes only one of the outcomes, the physical appearance. For all its successes, bariatric surgery does not attempt to change the cravings, binging, purging, and related problems, which are only corrected by getting the calcium, magnesium, and vitamin D components to their 90 percent reference level. The mood swings and fatigue drivers are only corrected with the rest of the WEE Protocol. This is the unfortunate truth. Many patients view surgery as an easy thing they can do. However, it does not require the actual behavioral changes and nutritional changes necessary for the overweight person to reach optimal health.

Thus, Sam, like many of our metabolic eating disorder patients, is always found to have other conditions related to metabolic eating disorders in various stages of development. I could recognize that Sam had several different metabolic eating disorders occurring at the same time, so he presented a unique challenge. This is not an uncommon situation in the WEE practice because each of these metabolic eating disorders comes from the same Cox-2 cytokine and the same calcium, magnesium, vitamin D, and vitamin B deficiencies. Carbohydrate excesses also require an insulin mimetic, cinnamon bark. Sam's metabolic eating disorders are all especially sensitive to his eating gluten-based carbohydrates and the toxic omega-6 fatty acids from seeds, nut, and their oils. The WEE Protocol was able to assist Sam in modifying his diet to correct the chemistry. This change made a difference in his hunger production caused by his metabolic eating disorder, which enabled him to continue responding to our nutritional therapy and gave him the energy to engage in his highly creative career.

When I began treating Sam, I had to better understand what had disabled his natural protection to allow him to get this particular disease condition in the first place. After I determined this, Sam and I worked the WEE Protocol to reverse his underlying chemistry in order to prevent the disease from returning. So far it appears to have prevented Sam from developing any new metabolic eating disorders, or other diseases for that matter.

Starting the WEE Protocol

The Wee Protocol consists of several essential clinical and education elements that are very important because the symptoms, their lab markers, and the disease itself can vary greatly in each patient. Another summary of the Wee Protocol follows for clarity.

STEP 1: *The introduction to WEE in nutrigenomics class, whether public or private, is an important place for patients, their families, and their supporters to start their road back to optimal health.* This class gives each a sense of the origin and evolution of the Western food supply or diet, its toxicities, deficiencies, and excesses contributing to their problems. The principles covered in this book form the basis of these classes. By reading this book, you've already taken the first step on the road to optimal health. However, if you are able to attend a class, you will still benefit from the in-person learning and the updates to what we've discovered since the book was published.

The WEE Protocol emphasizes the importance of and methods for determining the patient's change-operating system as well as that of the family and supporters since change is hard for each of us. The WEE Protocol, as well as the nutrigenomic nutrition lecture, reviews scientific articles and defines the differences between our human requirements and those of other mammals used in research, such as rats. This is known as the rat bias. While the rat bias is often hidden or completely overlooked in often-quoted nutritional research, this concept explains why products based on research with rats, such as drugs, nutrients, and even some health foods, do not work with or feel right to our human nutrigenomic systems.

The risk we run in depending on nonhuman research information gave rise to the WEE Protocol educational sessions. They are needed to better inform patients to protect them and their family and supporters from being distracted by outdated, disproven nutritional and health misinformation. Such misinformation often appears on television talk shows or in newsletters from disease-based associations or support groups. It even appears in newsletters that are alleged to be from institutions with credible-sounding names but that are not actually from those credible institutions.

STEP 2: *The patient meets with a trained WEE educator/provider.* This is a doctor or certified nurse practitioner (CNP) who is familiar with the WEE Protocol. This first visit is the WEE Protocol Intake. It usually focuses on the person's and/or family's current reasons and goals for nutrigenomic consultation and follow-up care, current diet and supplements, current symptoms, family history, and the WEE Protocol 90/360 Lab Assessment. The WEE Protocol Intake also covers current and past use of cosmetics and personal care supplies to determine if they contain toxic elements, such as gluten, heavy metals, and propylene glycol (i.e., antifreeze).

Step 2 also involves discussing the change readiness of the patient, family, and supporters present at the intake and the support systems in place to assist the patient and family in making those essential changes needed to absorb deficient elements and reduce toxic ones. Patients and their supporters are encouraged to discuss barriers to the changes needed along financial, cultural, educational, and personal lines, as well as insurance or resource limits for correlative lab testing.

STEP 3: *The physician's assessment of the patient leads to establishing an initial plan pending the results of the WEE Protocol 90/360 Lab Assessment.* This includes a review of the intake documentation and clinical assessment of deficiencies, toxicities, and findings related to lab results, if available. The physician then establishes start-up levels of nutrient options for the patient, including supplement dosages.

The 90/360 labs are ordered as covered by insurance to access the following toxicities:

- gluten effects on adrenals, bowels, the immune system, kidneys, liver, and the thyroid using the gliadin panel and HLA DQ 2,8 celiac gene typing or tissue transglutaminase (ttg) and endomysial antibody test, plus liver and renal function tests
- omega-6 fatty acid effects on bone marrow and body with complete blood count (CBC) and differential
- carbohydrate effects on the pancreas, thyroid, and liver with tests for HgbA1c, liver function, insulin, and C-peptide

The 90/360 labs are ordered as covered by insurance to access the following deficiencies:

- C-reactive protein to assess vitamin B complex and magnesium deficiencies and HDL for Vitamin B2 and magnesium deficiency
- calcium, magnesium, and vitamin D totals, intact parathyroid hormone (PTH), and total cholesterol and LDL for mineral deficiencies

The 90/360 labs are ordered as covered by insurance to assess functioning of:

- pituitary function is tested by looking at levels of adrenocorticotropic hormone (ACTH), follicle-stimulating hormone (FSH), luteinizing hormone (LH), plus thyroid-stimulating hormone (TSH), thyroid peroxidase (TPO), and parathyroid hormone (PTH)
- thyroid function is tested by looking at levels of TSH, TPO, triiodothyronine (T3), total thyroxine (T4), and free thyroxine (FTI)
- adrenal gland function is tested by looking at levels of cortisol and dehydroepiandrosterone hormones (DHEAs)

Levels of the following sex hormones are also tested: estradiol, estrone, enhanced estrogen, free testosterone, and total testosterone.

STEP 4: *The 90/360 Lab Assessment or more limited lab results are combined with the original physician assessment to set the specific nutrigenomic plan and protocol for the patient's next thirty to one-hundred twenty days.* The next steps then vary depending on the patient's status and needs. Options include:

- a thirty-day abnormal lab reassessment is followed by a physician/CNP visit if patient's condition is terminal or critical or if the patient desires to move forward on the plan more quickly.
- a sixty-to-one-hundred twenty-day abnormal lab reassessment followed by a physician/CNP visit provides a progressive review and plan adjustment for those more concerned with improvements moving along in a steady timeline.
- ninety to one-hundred twenty-day abnormal lab reassessment followed by a physician/CNP visit provides maximum improvement at less cost over a longer timeline, yet without a plateau effect.

- greater than one-hundred twenty-day abnormal lab reassessment is NOT recommended since performance will plateau after 120 days without additional changes made based on lab assessments and symptom assessments.
- a nonregular reassessment plan is reserved for out–of-state or out-of-country patients as well as those patients who request it for personal, financial, or insurance reasons.

The lab assessment, plan preparation, and ongoing follow-up have been standardized to ensure that the protocol is followed in the manner in which it was developed and in the format in which it has had predictable, reliable outcomes for more than 32,000 patient encounters/visits.

At the same time, the concept is personalized so you, the patient, can get the elements in the manner that best suits your learning and functioning. In the beginning and at the end, you, the patient, and your family and supporters are the ones making all the decisions that suit your lifestyle and the outcomes you desire to achieve. The WEE Protocol simply provides the methods to help you achieve those outcomes.

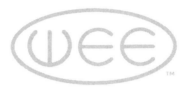

RESOURCES FOR LIFE— FOR THE REST OF YOUR LIFE

The following pages contain nutritional tools we use with our patients, as well as references for further reading. They are meant to guide you as you work your side of the WEE Protocol. They will help you select better foods and plan meals at home and at restaurants.

I've also included a section for you to use with your doctor to plan your doses of supplements using the simple yet effective computations I have used for more than 32,000 patient visits. Of course it would be easier if we, or your doctor, worked through this with you.

The charts that follow are a list of foods that give you a positive balance of omega-3 fatty acids or that are easily balanced with triple strength fish oil. I've also included information about

Healthful Foods to Decrease Omega-6 Fatty Acids and Increase Complex Carbohydrates*				
	omega-6 (mg)	omega-3 (mg)	Positive Balance (mg)	Glycemic Load
Vegetables (1/2 cup)				
Brussels sprouts	60	131	71	2
Broccoli	17	57	40	1
Cauliflower	12	38	26	1
Lettuce (loose leaf)	13	32	19	1
Turnips	8	26	18	3
Boston lettuce	9	23	14	1
Kale (raw)	46	60	14	1
Spinach (raw)	3	17	14	0
Romaine lettuce	9	21	12	1
Zucchini	14	23	9	1
Radish	9	17	8	1
Crookneck squash	12	20	8	1
Acorn squash	11	20	8	1
Green beans	13	20	7	1
Wax beans	13	20	7	1
Cucumber	16	22	6	1
Cabbage	18	23	5	1
Pumpkin	1	2	1	3

Healthful Foods to Decrease Omega-6 Fatty Acids and Increase Complex Carbohydrates*				
	omega-6 (mg)	omega-3 (mg)	Positive Balance (mg)	Glycemic Load
Beans (1 cup)				
Kidney beans (canned)	187	297	110	4
Pinto beans (canned)	293	401	108	4
Meats (3 oz portion)				
Wild-caught salmon	373	1786	1413	0
omega-3 eggs	40	600	560	0
Sardine (per 1, not in oil)	184	739	555	0
Shrimp	98	464	366	0
Crab	54	402	348	0
Tuna (water-packed)	37	250	213	0
Perch	24	69	45	0
Fruit (1 cup)				
Papaya nectar**	18	70	52	15
Papaya**	14	58	44	10
Mangoes**	23	61	38	8
Cantaloupe**	26	35	9	4
Honeydew**	21	28	7	4
Cheese (1 oz)				
Gouda	75	112	35	0
Roquefort	175	200	25	0
Parmesan	90	98	8	0
Romano	81	88	2	0

* Patients with metabolic disorder, hypertension, low HDL, high triglycerides, or high cholesterol or LDL, or obesity, diabetes, polycystic ovarian syndrome, or cancer should keep their glycemic load less than 100 per day and/or use cinnamon to compensate for extra carbohydrates.

** Fruits should be naturally ripened and eaten in season or purchased canned or frozen out of season to avoid latex complications.

Healthful Foods That Are Easily Balanced to Decrease Omega-6 Fatty Acids and Increase Complex Carbohydrates				
	omega-6 (mg)	omega-3 (mg)	Positive Balance (mg)	Glycemic Load
Cereals/Grains (1 cup)				
Wild rice	195	156	-39	18
Rice Chex	58	11	-47	23
White rice (medium grain)	86	19	-67	23
Corn Chex	99	3	-96	21
Corn flakes	109	3	-106	24
Rice Krispies	144	31	-113	22
Crispix	113	3	-110	22
Cream of rice	192	42	-150	22
Grits (⅓ cup in 1⅓ cup water)	252	5	-247	9
Brown rice	603	27	-576	16
Vegetables (1/2 cup)				
Potato	12	4	-8	26
Sweet potato	34	6	-28	21
Artichoke	41	15	-26	3
Onion	34	2	-32	2
Eggplant	39	7	-32	2
Beets	38	3	-35	5
Carrots	41	6	-35	3
Asparagus	56	3	-53	3
Peppers	69	7	-62	1
Peas	110	25	-85	3
Tomatoes	234	9	-225	3
Lima beans	120	57	-63	12
Corn	291	9	-292	11

Healthful Foods That Are Easily Balanced to Decrease Omega-6 Fatty Acids and Increase Complex Carbohydrates				
	omega-6 (mg)	omega-3 (mg)	Positive Balance (mg)	Glycemic Load
Beans (1 cup)				
Great Northern	182	149	-33	7
Navy beans	244	204	-40	7
Black beans	322	270	-52	7
Breads (1 slice/item)				
Brown-rice bread	447	29	-418	8
Meat (3 oz serving)				
New Zealand lamb	536	340	-196	0
Steak (porterhouse)	273	51	-222	0
Ground beef (1 patty)	293	43	-250	0
Pork chop	816	26	-790	0
Fruit (1/2 cup)				
Orange (1 small)	17	7	-10	5
Apple (1 small)	92	19	-73	5
Cheese/Dairy (1 oz)				
Cottage cheese (4 oz)	47	19	-28	0
Cheddar	164	103	-61	0
Bleu	152	75	-77	0

the glycemic load and serving sizes for each food item. *Keep in mind that if you are sensitive to any of the foods listed, you should not include them in your diet, even if they are good for omega-3: omega-6 balance.* For additional help in managing your omega-3:omega-6 balance, use the KIM-2, Keep It Managed program, from the National Institutes of Health (NIH) to track your foods. See: *http://EFAeducation.nih.gov.*

Next are some suggestions for low-glycemic, omega-balanced meals to be eaten out or cooked at home. The glycemic index values for each meal listed are all less than 10.

Remember to obtain an omega balance by eating as closely as possible to the 1:1 ratio and supplementing with triple strength fish oil to make up the difference. Omega fatty acid counts are estimated in the menus that follow. Exact amounts will vary depending on the items chosen, including fruits and vegetables.

Meal and Snack Recommendations

BREAKFAST

Smoothie made with whey protein, milk, and fruit
- Omega-6: 235 mg
- Omega-3: 155 mg
- Balance: -80 mg

1 oz cheese and 1 cup fruit or vegetables
- Omega-6: 328 mg
- Omega-3: 222 mg
- Balance: -106 mg

BREAKFAST (cont'd)

1 cup yogurt with 1 cup fruit
or vegetables
- Omega-6: 387 mg
- Omega-3: 209 mg
- Balance: -209 mg

2 links sausage with 1 cup fruit
or vegetable
- Omega-6: 1064
- Omega-3: 203
- Balance: -861

1 cup pinto beans
with 2 slices Canadian bacon
- Omega-6: 457
- Omega-3: 242
- Balance: −215

Simple Shopping List to Stock Your Refrigerator and Pantry with WEE-Friendly Foods

Rice

Rice and corn cereals

Rice cakes

Rice or potato bread

Milk

Yogurt

Cheese

Butter

Ice cream (not artificially sweetened or low fat)

Eggs

Bacon

Sausage (make sure it does not contain MSG)

Fruit (in-season or canned/frozen)

Vegetables (in-season or canned/frozen)

Lettuce

Coffee

Tea

Beans (dried or canned)

Meats low in omega-6

Potatoes

Popcorn (air-popped)

LUNCH/DINNER

Wild-caught salmon
with 1 cup fruit or vegetable

- Omega-6: 618
- Omega-3: 1,903
- Balance +1,285

New Zealand lamb
with 1 cup fruit or vegetable
Omega-6: 586
Omega-3: 303
Balance −286

Shrimp stir-fry with vegetables
and 1 teaspoon butter

- Omega-6: 264
- Omega-3: 394
- Balance +49

1 cup chili with 1 tablespoon
sour cream

- Omega-6: 589
- Omega-3: 429
- Balance −160

Shrimp stir-fry with vegetables
(1 teaspoon olive oil)

- Omega-6: 516
- Omega-3: 366
- Balance −150

1 cup beef stew with 1 cup fruit
or vegetable

- Omega-6: 426
- Omega-3: 283
- Balance −143

Tuna salad (made with sour
cream or yogurt instead of
mayonnaise) with lettuce

- Omega-6: 157
- Omega-3: 618
- Balance +461

Roast beef lettuce wrap
with tomato and cream cheese

- Omega-6: 345
- Omega-3: 178
- Balance −167

LUNCH/DINNER

Ham lettuce wrap with cheese, tomato, and cream cheese

- Omega-6: 549
- Omega-3: 202
- Balance −347

Pork loin and 1 cup fruit or vegetable

- Omega-6: 1181
- Omega-3: 51
- Balance −1,031

Hamburger (no bun)
with 1 cup fruit or vegetable

- Omega-6: 475
- Omega-3: 117
- Balance −358

RECIPE IDEAS FOR CONDIMENTS

Creamy dressings

Greek or plain yogurt with vinegar or lemon juice, feta or gorgonzola cheese, fresh chives and other spices, instead of mayonnaise.

Ranch or bleu cheese dressing made with buttermilk, cottage cheese, or sour cream.

Vinaigrette dressings

Combine olive oil sparingly, vinegar, lemon juice, crushed raspberries, honey, and season with garlic, salt, pepper, or other herb and spice combinations.

Vegetable dips

Blend sour cream and cream cheese with lemon juice, grated onion, fresh chives, sundried tomatoes, and other spices.

Bean dip (similar to hummus)

Blend pinto or black beans, roasted garlic, lemon or lime juice, and spices.

SNACKS

In-season fresh vegetables and Greek yogurt dip

In-season fresh vegetables and bean spread (pinto beans and roasted garlic)

Sardines, herring, or anchovies

Hard-boiled eggs

Dried meats such as jerky, pepperoni, and prosciutto

Yogurt, cottage cheese, or cheese slices

Shrimp cocktail

Additional information about the omega fatty acid makeup of foods can be found in the KIM-2 system at *efaeducation.nih.gov*.

The following recommendations will assist in selection of proteins, cooking oils, fruits, and vegetables:

Proteins: Dairy, eggs, and beans can be eaten daily. Meats low in omega-6 such as beef, lamb, pork, or wild-caught fish can be eaten weekly if you are not vegetarian.

Cooking Oils: Lard and butter are best; use clarified butter such as ghee if using butter at higher temperatures. Extra virgin olive oil is satisfactory when used sparingly. Extra virgin olive oil sprayed from a bottle onto vegetables just before stir-frying decreases smoking.

Fruits: In-season fruits are best when available. Canned or frozen fruits are best if not in season in your location to reduce the latex content.

Vegetables: Choose a variety of colored vegetables, including yellow, red, white, orange, and green. Eating stalks and root vegetables improves alkaline content.

Your NutriGenomic-Focused Protocol Worksheet

1. Look yourself over for signs of deficiency and use your lab results to calculate supplement dosages.
2. Consult with your doctor for a complete history and physical exam.
3. Begin your nutrigenomic dietary regimen based on your lab results and clinical findings. Begin an omega-6 fatty acid reduced diet to enhance the effect of added omega-3 if your monocyte count is greater than 5 percent and/or add four triple strength fish oil capsules for each percent over 5 percent **if approved by your physician**.
   - If your C-reactive protein is greater than zero, add one time-released B-100 for each 0.50 up to a total of six tablets per day taken before meals **if approved by your physician**.
   - If tumor markers are elevated, add four more triple strength fish oil capsules daily **if approved by your physician**.
   - Begin a glycemic-reduced diet if your International Classification

of Glycemic Index load is greater than 100 and your:

+ HDL is less than 60, and add one timed-release B-100 vitamin complex tablet for each 0.50 up to six tablets per day taken with meals **if approved by your physician.**

+ HgbA1c is greater than 5.8, and add four cinnamon bark 500-mg capsules for each 0.1 elevation over 5.8 up to sixteen tablets per day taken before meals, snacks, and bedtime **if approved by your physician.**

+ Triglycerides are greater than 100, and add four cinnamon bark 500-mg capsules for each 50 mg/dl over 100 up to sixteen tablets per day taken before meals, snacks, and bedtime **if approved by your physician.**

■ Begin gluten-reduced diet if TPO is great than 0 and/or HLA DQ 2,8 celiac typing gene pair is present. Redouble your efforts to remove gluten if antigliadin antibodies are greater than 1.0 **if approved by your physician.**

4. Attend workshops with a WEE educator at two, six, ten, and fourteen weeks.

■ Review effectiveness of the patient in maintaining the dietary interventions.

■ Diet reinforcement using the KIM-2 program at *http://EFA-education.nih.gov.*

■ Diet reinforcement to maintain a glycemic load of less than 100 using the International Classification of Glycemic Index.

Follow-up Labs and Visit Schedule

Schedule follow-up labs and visits four, eight, twelve, and sixteen weeks after beginning the WEE Protocol. Have your labs drawn the week prior to your appointment so that you will have the results for your appointment. Review progress, diet, symptoms, CT scans and MRI reports, and biomarkers, as appropriate.

Use the following labs and results to adjust your supplement dosages with your physician:

- Monocyte count used to adjust omega-3 fish oil level
- C-reactive protein level used to adjust the B-complex dose
- HDL level used to adjust the B complex, cinnamon, and magnesium levels
- HbgA1c level used to adjust the B complex, cinnamon, and magnesium levels
- Magnesium, calcium, vitamin D, and intact PTH level used to adjust magnesium oxide, calcium carbonate, and vitamin D3 levels

Labs will also help you and your health care provider to:

- review effectiveness of the patient in maintaining the dietary interventions.
- reinforce omega-6 dietary changes using the KIM-2 program at *http://etaeducation.nih.gov.*
- reinforce dietary changes to maintain glycemic index of less than 100 using the International Classification of Glycemic Index.

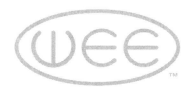

FURTHER READING

Introduction to the WEE Protocol

Cordain, L.; Eaton, S.B.; Sebastian, A.; Mann, N.; Lindeberg, S.; Watkins, B.A.; O'Keefe, J.H.; and Brand-Miller, J. "Origins and Evolution of the Western Diet: Health Implications for the 21st Century." *American Journal of Clinical Nutrition* 81, no. 2 (February 2005): 341–54. This article discusses the change from simple nutrition that was stable for thousands and thousands of years before modern agribusiness and transportation changes impacted the foods available and the movement of peoples. *www.ncbi.nlm.nih.gov/pubmed/15699220*

Contributions to Modern Illness

Arentz-Hansen, H.; Fleckenstein, B.; Molberg, Ø.; Scott, H.; Koning, F.; Jung, G.; Roepstorff, P.; Lundin K. E.; Sollid, L.M. "The molecular basis for oat intolerance in patients with celiac disease." *PLoS Medicine.* 2004.

Blanco, C.; Carrillo, T.; Castillo, R., et al. "Latex Allergy: Clinical Features and Cross-Reactivity with Fruits." *Annals of Allergy* 73 (1994): 309–14. An abstract of this article is given at two Web sites. *anaphylacticreactions. com/latexdisplay.asp?num=14* and *www.latexallergyresources.org/File-Downloads/Latex-food%20cross-reactivity%20review.pdf*

Cheng, X.; Shi, H.; Adams, C.D.; Ma, Y. "Assessment of Metal Contamina-
    tions Leaching Out from Recycling Plastic Bottles upon Treatments."
    Environmental Science and Pollution Research International. 17, no. 7
    (August 17, 2010):1323–30. ePub: 2010 Mar 23.

Cunha, N.V.; de Abreu, S.B.; Panis, C.; Grassiolli, S. ; Guarnier, F.A.; Cecchini,
    R.; Mazzuco, T.L.; Pinge-Filho, P.; and Martins-Pinge, M.C. "Cox-2
    Inhibition Attenuates Cardiovascular and Inflammatory Aspects in
    Monosodium Glutamate-induced Obese Rats." *Life Sciences.* 87, no.
    11–12 (September 11, 2010): 375–381. The abstract of this article is avail-
    able at no cost at the publisher's Web site at *www.sciencedirect.com/
    science/article/pii/S0024320510003346*

Davis, Donald R.; Epp, Melvin D.; and Riordan, Hugh D. "Changes in USDA
    Food Composition Data for 43 Garden Crops, 1950 to 1999." *Journal of
    the American College of Nutrition* 23, no. 6 (December 2004): 669-682.
    www.jacn.org/cgi/content/abstract/23/6/669

Friedman, M. "Nutritional Consequences of Food Processing." *Forum Nutrition.*
    56 (2003): 350–2. The author is from the Western Regional Research
    Center, Agricultural Research Service, USDA, Albany, California
    94710.

Hoozemans, J.J.; Veerhuis, R.; Rozemuller, A.J.; and Eikelenboom, P. "The
    Pathological Cascade of Alzheimer's Disease: The Role of Inflam-
    mation and its Therapeutic Implications." *Drugs of Today.* 38, no. 6
    (June 2002): 429–43. This scientific article at the National Center for
    Biotechnical Information Web site describes a cascade of Alzheimer's
    disease, including the role of inflammation and implications for thera-
    peutic treatment. *www.ncbi.nlm.nih.gov/pubmed/12532179*

Jiménez-Monreal, A.M.; García-Diz, L.; Martínez-Tomé, M.; Mariscal, M.; Mur-
    cia, M.A. "Influence of Cooking Methods on Antioxidant Activity of
    Vegetables." *Journal of Food Science.* 74, no. 3 (April 2009): H97–H103.

Lim, D.S.; Kwack, S.J.; Kim, K.B.; Kim, H.S.; Lee, B.M. "Potential Risk of Bisphenol
    A Migration from Polycarbonate Containers after Heating, Boiling, and
    Microwaving." *Journal of Toxicology and Environmental Health.* 72, no.
    21–22 (2009): 1285–91.

Liu, L.; Jiang Z; Huang X; Liu J; Zhang J; Xiao J; Bao Q; Wen J; Zhang S; Zhu D;
    Zhang P; Zhang L. Jiangsu. "Disappearance of Sexual Dimorphism in
    Triptolide Metabolism in Monosodium Glutamate Treated Neonatal
    Rats." *Arzneimittel-Forschung.* 61, no. 2 (2011): 98–103.

Roman-Ramos, R.; Almanza-Perez, J.C.; Garcia-Macedo, R.; Blancas-Flores, G.;
    Fortis-Barrera, A.; Jasso, E.I.; Garcia-Lorenzana, M.; Campos-Sepul-
    veda, A.E.; Cruz, M.; Alarcon-Aguilar, F.J. "Monosodium Glutamate
    Neonatal Intoxication Associated with Obesity in Adult Stage Is Char-

acterized by Chronic Inflammation and Increased mRNA Expression of Peroxisome Proliferator-Activated Receptors in Mice." *Basic & Clinical Pharmacology & Toxicology*. 108, no. 6 (June 2011): 406-413. The abstract of this article is available at no cost at the publisher's Web site at: *onlinelibrary.wiley.com/doi/10.1111/j.1742-7843.2011.00671.x/abstract*

Yuan, Y.; Chen, F.; Zhao, G.H.; Liu, J.; Zhang, H.X.; Hu, X.S. "A Comparative Study of Acrylamide Formation Induced by Microwave and Conventional Heating Methods." *Journal of Food Science* 72, no. 4 (May 2007): C212–6.

Fixing It

Balanzá-Martinez V.; Fries G.R.; Colpo G.D.; Silveira P.P.; et al. "Therapeutic use of omega-3 fatty acids in bipolar disorder." *Expert Review of Neurotherapeutics*. 2011 Jul;11(7):1029–47.

Berquin I.M.; Edwards I.J.; Chen Y.Q. "Multi-targeted therapy of cancer by omega-3 fatty acids." *Cancer Letters*. 2008 Oct 8;269(2):363–77. Epub 2008 May 13. Review.

Chapkin R.S.; Seo J.; McMurray D.N.; Lupton J.R. "Mechanisms by which docosahexaenoic acid and related fatty acids reduce colon cancer risk and inflammatory disorders of the intestine." *Chemistry and Physics of Lipids*. 2008 May;153(1):14–23. Epub 2008 Mar 4. Review.

Delattre A.M.; et al. "Evaluation of chronic omega-3 fatty acids supplementation on behavioral and neurochemical alterations in 6-hydroxydopamine-lesion model of Parkinson's disease." *Neuroscience Research*. 2010 Mar;66(3):256–64. Epub 2009 Nov 24.

Dupertuis Y.M.; Meguid M.M.; Pichard C. "Colon cancer therapy: new perspectives of nutritional manipulations using polyunsaturated fatty acids." *Current Opinion in Nutrition & Metabolic Care*. 2007 Jul;10(4):427–32. Review.

Gillet L.; Roger S.; Bougnoux P.; LeGuennec J.Y.; Besson P. "Beneficial effects of omega-3 long-chain fatty acids in breast cancer and cardiovascular diseases: voltage-gated sodium channels as a common feature?" *Biochimie*. 2011 Jan;93(1):4–6. Epub 2010 Feb 16. Review.

Jia W.; Slominski B.A.; Guenter W.; Humphreys A.; Jones O. "The effect of enzyme supplementation on egg production parameters and omega-3 fatty acid deposition in laying hens fed flaxseed and canola seed." *Poultry Science*. 2008 Oct;87(10):2005–14.

Kew S.; Banerjee T.; Minihane A.M.; Finnegan Y.E.; et al. "Relation between the fatty acid composition of peripheral blood mononuclear cells and measures of immune cell function in healthy, free-living subjects aged 25–72 y." *American Journal of Clinical Nutrition*. 2003 May;77(5):1278–86.

Larsson S.C.; Kumlin M.; Ingelman-Sunberg M.; Wolk A. "Dietary long-chain n-3 fatty acids for the prevention of cancer: a review of potential mechanisms." *American Journal of Clinincal Nutrition.* 2004 Jun;79(6):935–45.

Martins J.G. "EPA but not DHA appears to be responsible for the efficacy of omega-3 long chain polyunsaturated fatty acid supplementation in depression: evidence from a meta-analysis of RCTs." *Journal of the American College of Nutrition.* 2009 Oct;28(5):525–42.

Patterson R.E.; Flatt S.W.; Newman V.A.; Natarajan, Rock C.L.; Thomson C.A.; Caan B.J., et al. "Marine fatty acid intake is associated with breast cancer prognosis." *Journal of Nutrition.* 2011 Feb;141(2):201–6.

Pauwels E.K.; Kairemo K. "Fatty acid facts, part II: role in the prevention of carcinogenesis, or, more fish on the dish?" *Drug News Perspect.* 2008 Nov;21(9):504–10. Review.

Reese A.C.; Fradet V.; Witte J.S. "Omega-3 fatty acids, genetic variants in cox-2 and prostate cancer." *Journal of Nutrigent and Nutrigenomics.* 2009.

Saugstad L.F.. "Infantile autism: a chronic psychosis since infancy due to synaptic pruning of the supplementary motor area." *Nutrition and Health.* 2008 Mar;19(4):307–17.

Theis F.; et al. "Dietary supplementation with eicosapentaenoic acid, but not with other long-chain n-3 or n-6 polyunsaturated fatty acids, decreases natural killer cell activity in healthy subjects aged >55y." *American Journal of Clinincal Nutrition.* 2001 Mar;73(3):539–48.

Thiébaut A.C.; Chajès V., Gerber M.; Boutron-Ruault M.C.; Joulin V.; Lenoir G.; Berrino F.; Riboli E.; Bénichou J.; Clavel-Chapelon F. "Dietary intakes of omega-6 and omega-3 polyunsaturated fatty acids and the risk of breast cancer." *International Journal of Cancer.* 2009 Feb 15;124(4):924–31.

Venna V.R.; et al. "PUFA induce antidepressant-like effects in parallel to structural and molecular changes in the hippocampus." *Psychoneuroendocrinology.* 2009 Feb;34(2):199–211.

Wall R.; Ross R.P.; Fitzgerald G.F.; Stanton C. "Fatty acids from fish: the anti-inflammatory potential of long-chain omega-3 fatty acids." *Nutrition Reviews.* May;68(5):280–9. Review.

For clarity with Figure 7, here are some definitions:

angiogenesis: the formation of new blood vessels, particularly in the case of those vessels that are formed to help feed a tumor. In the diagram following, we are talking about angiogenesis in the context of cancer, so in this instance, the formation of new blood vessels occurs to support a tumor.

tumor-endothelial cell adhesion: the attachment of tumor cells to endothelial cells (those cells that line blood vessels, lymph vessels, etc.). This adhesion plays a role in the spread of cancer as tumors and cancer cells attach to endothelial cells.

reactive oxygen species: a type of molecule (including hydrogen peroxide and hydroxyl radical) containing oxygen, which may be important to cell signaling at low levels, but at high levels, they may be implicated in cell damage and programmed cell death.

reactive nitrogen species: a type of molecule that contains nitrogen, reacts easily with other molecules, and may be implicated in cell damage.

ROS and **NOS** are both the types of molecules that antioxidants help to fight against.

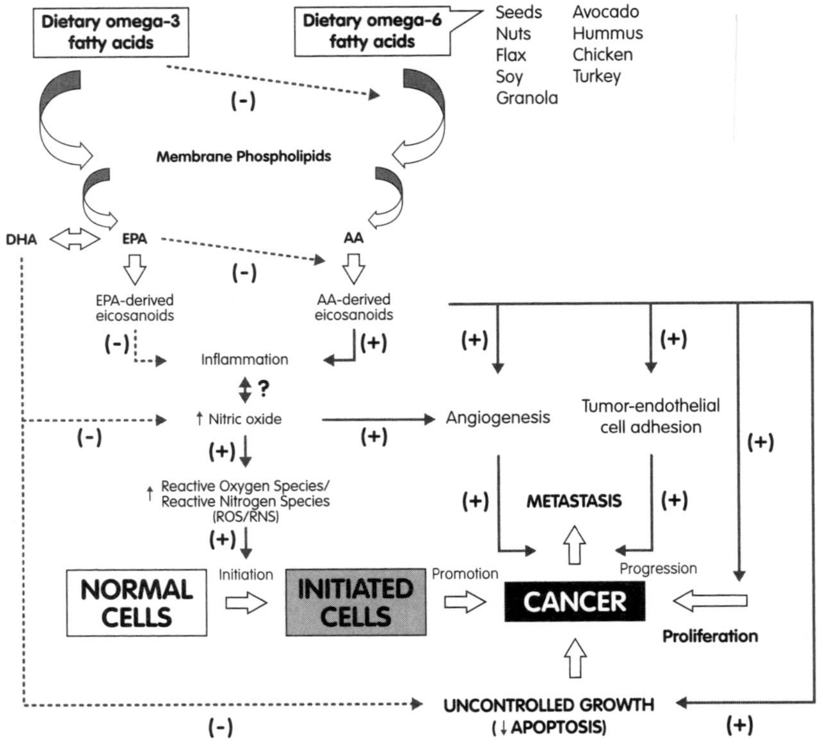

Dietary omega-3 fatty acids

Dietary omega-6 fatty acids

Seeds · Avocado
Nuts · Hummus
Flax · Chicken
Soy · Turkey
Granola

(−)

Membrane Phospholipids

DHA ⟺ EPA ---- AA

(−)

EPA-derived eicosanoids

AA-derived eicosanoids

(−) Inflammation (+)

↕ ?

↑ Nitric oxide → Angiogenesis

(−) (+)

(+) ↓

↑ Reactive Oxygen Species/ Reactive Nitrogen Species (ROS/RNS)

(+) ↓

(+) (+)

Tumor-endothelial cell adhesion

(+) METASTASIS (+)

(+)

NORMAL CELLS → Initiation → INITIATED CELLS → Promotion → CANCER ⟸ Proliferation

Progression

(−) UNCONTROLLED GROWTH (↓ APOPTOSIS) (+)

Figure 7. *This figure represents my adaptation from a simplified version of the cytokine pathways resulting when humans eat omega-3 and omega-6 fatty acids in their diets. If the path of each type of fatty acid is followed, the omega-3 fatty acids are seen to decrease, or have a negative effect, on inflammation and unregulated cell growth (i.e., cancer). However, omega-6 fatty acids increase, or have a positive effect, on inflammation, reactive oxygen species and reactive nitrogen species (ROS/RNS), angiogenesis, and tumor-endothelial cell adhesion, which lead to metastasizing cancers.*

Source: Larsson, Susanna C., *et al.* "Dietary long-chain n–3 fatty acids for the prevention of cancer." *American Journal of Clinical Nutrition.* 79, no. 6 (June 2004): 935–45. The National Institute of Environmental Medicine, Karolinska Institutet, Stockholm.

Author Note: While the example is displayed for cancer, similar models have been developed for neurological, autoimmune, metabolic, and pain syndromes.

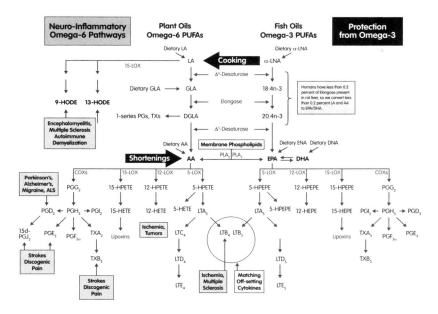

Figure 8. *An overview of metabolism in the human body of omega-6 plant oil and omega-3 polyunsaturated fatty acids (PUFAs) into eicosanoids, which are cellular chemicals involved in inflammation and neuroinflammation. The names of these eicosanoids are in bold and are detailed as follows: LA, linoleic acid (18:2n–6); -LNA, -linolenic acid (18:3n–3); GLA, -linolenic acid (18:3n–6); DGLA, dihomo- -linolenic acid (20:3n–6); AA, arachidonic acid (20:4n–6); EPA, eicosapentaenoic acid (20:5n–3); DHA, docosahexaenoic acid (22:6n–3); PLA2, phospholipase A2; LOX, lipoxygenase; COXs, cyclooxygenases (COX-1 and COX-2); 15-HETE, 15(S)-hydroxyeicosatetraenoic acid; 12-HETE, 12-hydroxyeicosatetraenoic acid; 5-HETE, 5-hydroxyeicosatetraenoic acid; HEPE, hydroxyeicosapentaenoic acid; HPETE, hydroperoxyeicosatetraenoic acid; HPEPE, hydroperoxyeicosapentaenoic acid; LT, leukotriene; HODE, hydroxyoctadecadienoic acid; PG, prostaglandin; TX, thromboxane.*

Source: Larsson, Susanna C., *et al.* "Dietary long-chain n–3 fatty acids for the prevention of cancer." *American Journal of Clinical Nutrition.* 79, no. 6 (June 2004): 935–45. The National Institute of Environmental Medicine, Karolinska Institutet, Stockholm.

For further reading about human genetic markers, major histo-compatibility complex/genetics pedigree, genetic polymorphism, and disease susceptibility, see *www.ncbi.nlm.nih.gov/pubmed/9192057*

About the Author

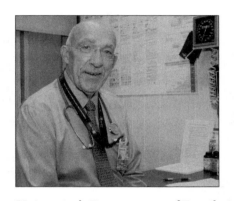

Dr. Glen Aukerman is Professor of Family Medicine at The Ohio State University in Columbus, Ohio, where he serves as Medical Director of the University's Center of Integrative Medicine. Dr. Aukerman has also served as Chair of The Ohio State University's Department of Family Medicine and as President of the American Academy of Family Physicians. His articles have appeared in *American Family Physician*, *The Journal of the American Medical Association (JAMA)*, *The Journal of Family Practice*, and *The Ohio Family Physician*. He is also a contributor to *Saunders Manual of Family Practice* and a reviewer for *Family Practice Research Journal*. He is the recipient of the Distinguished Service Award from the Ohio Academy of Family Physicians Foundation, the Clinical Excellence Award from The Ohio State University Medical Center, and The Ohio State University College of Nursing Individual Health Education Award. Prior to his distinguished career at Ohio State, Dr. Aukerman held medical teaching posts at West Virginia University and the University of Tennessee-Memphis, and also served as Deputy Director and Chief Medical Officer at the U.S. Health Resources and Services Administration's National Practitioner Data Bank.